POSITIVE LIVES
Responses to HIV

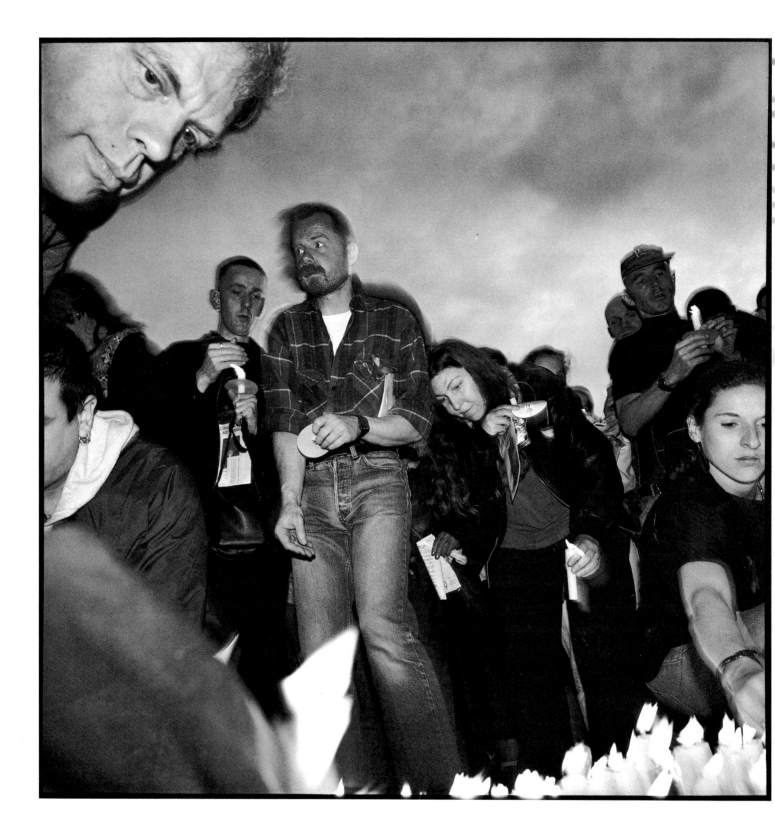

POSITIVE LIVES

Responses to HIV

A PHOTODOCUMENTARY

Edited by Stephen Mayes, *Network Photographers,*
and Lyndall Stein, *The Terrence Higgins Trust*

CASSELL

The Cassell AIDS Awareness Series also includes
How Can You Write a Poem When You're Dying of AIDS?
(edited by John Harold)

Cassell
Villiers House, 41/47 Strand
London WC2N 5JE

387 Park Avenue South
New York, NY 10016-8810

First published 1993

BRITISH LIBRARY CATALOGUING-IN-PUBLICATION DATA
A catalogue record for this book is available from the British Library.

LIBRARY OF CONGRESS CATALOGING-IN-PUBLICATION DATA
A catalogue record for this book is available from the Library of Congress.

ISBN 0-304-32846-4

Designed and typeset by Ronald Clark
Printed and bound in Great Britain by
Butler & Tanner Limited, Frome

CONTENTS

FOREWORD

Today, people are so afraid of dying that they've decided only those with AIDS will die. There's a line in a decadent French novel, 'As for living, our servants can do that for us.' The contemporary version seems to be, 'As for dying, all those strange, marginal, "at-risk" groups can do that for us.'

These photographs show that everyone is at risk. Those with HIV are not just crowded into the margins but are also inscribed in what printers call the 'body text', the main blocks of type in the book of our lives. These photographs are powerful, and they systematically disabuse us of our ready-made clichés, those mental pictures in which we never appear.

Here are not just isolated individuals but couples embracing on a hospital bed in the presence of the patient's parents. Here we see not only prisoners but also children, not just patients but also buddies, friends, doctors – even a nurse so tense that she needs a session of shiatsu massage. Memories of adventures past are invoked but so are the erotic present and the fearful future.

I've thought hard about how to live in the present. My lover (who is French) has AIDS and I've been HIV-positive since at least 1985 – the first moment when the test to detect the virus became available. Soon after he was diagnosed at the end of 1989, we moved to the United States for a year, but whilst we were there he was unable to work as an architect (no jobs to be had). He took up a new career as a cartoonist. As he's a perfectionist, he worked night and day on his drawings for a year before he showed them to anyone. With amazing rapidity he evolved a style of his own, but he was constantly anxious; partly because he's always been consumed with self-doubt despite his remarkable successes, and partly because he knew he was on a very tight schedule. His life expectancy is far from brilliant. Yet despite the demands of his elegant style and his high standards, he's managed to produce one book of cartoons and is now planning another. I wonder how many of his laughing readers realize that many of these drawings were done while he was blind in one eye from herpes or fighting to regain his mental sharpness after a terrifying, disorienting bout of toxoplasmosis.

His real courage is to have taken up a new artistic pursuit at all. Naturally, on some level of awareness, everyone knows that all human efforts are futile or at least evanescent, but most of us manage to bury that appalling reality beneath the drudgery of work or the habitual routine of daily life. The person with AIDS, however, sees through necessity to the end of all needs – death. This vision neutralizes everything that is cosy, familiar and automatic. Someone once said that we couldn't go on living if we knew the moment of our death. AIDS gives us that tragic certainty. If we do go on living, it's out of either courage or purest folly – in spite of an acute awareness of existentialist absurdity.

Just as medieval monks contemplated human skulls in order to remind themselves of what lies in wait for all living creatures, in the same spirit the man or woman or child with AIDS never forgets for long the imminent approach of mortality. Periodic crises and the death of friends are potent reminders.

But what to do with this awareness? When my best friend died of AIDS I watched him in his last days juggle with two different senses of time, as though he were keeping two different sets of books on future accounts. He was intermittently lucid, knowing that all his efforts would soon be cut short; he wrote his will, saw friends, eliminated fools and finished his last book. At other times, however, he'd forget about his imminent death and would talk as most people do about projects five, ten or fifteen years hence. He was performing a delicate balancing act – fooling himself just enough to remain cheerfully engaged with the future, while being honest enough not to miss a second of the present. Our present which may be the only heaven we'll ever know – the heaven of friendship, of natural and artistic beauty, the ache of sensuality, the ennoblement of love, the taste of raspberries and cream.

Photography, as Roland Barthes observed, is always about death, since it records unrepeatable moments, captures the passing of the present and arrests that process of decay called time. The German poet Rilke went further when he wrote that whilst he, as a young man, held a sepia-tinted photograph of his father as a young cadet, he recognized that, not only was his father long since dead, but he himself was gliding steadily towards death – and the photograph was fading.

Each of the photographs in this exhibition is a *memento mori*, even as they are also reminders of all those unexpectedly joyful instants afforded by AIDS: the permission to be as different from the others as one has always longed to be; the courage to comfort the ill even in the cold heart of institutions (prison, hospital); the inspiration to devise new ways of expressing either faith or grief or to return to ways consecrated by tradition.

AIDS is a lonely thing. The body is alone and the mind fearful when one awakens at three in the morning, sheets drenched through with night sweats. AIDS is a despairing thing. It is a slow decomposition rather than a mercifully sudden surcease; it's a way of wearing down moral resistance, the devotion of friends, funds and resolutions to be optimistic. AIDS may be opportunistic, but it usually comes inopportunely to cut short lives that have yet to be fulfilled.

Nothing can eradicate this suffering, but an institution such as the Terrence Higgins Trust is a community and one that helps – with legal, medical and financial counsel, with information about treatment or resources, with everyday tasks such as shopping, cleaning, dressing and going out for a walk. AIDS is happening to us all, as these pictures show. I long for a miracle to eliminate the need for the Trust, but barring that, I hope everyone will contribute money and time.

Edmund White

PREFACE

The year 1993 marks the tenth anniversary of the Terrence Higgins Trust and the first decade of the AIDS epidemic in Britain. In that period the 'shape' of the epidemic has changed and its effects on a wide variety of communities have become more apparent.

This book dramatically illustrates some of the effects of HIV infection, on the lives of both individuals and communities. The photographs and the text record the crises, the grief and the loss brought by AIDS. However, they also show the courage of people with HIV and AIDS and the commitment of those working to counter the effects of the virus.

As chair of the Trust I see daily instances of the work done by volunteers and professionals to help relieve the effects of the epidemic. As someone who has had AIDS for five years I also respond to these photographs on a more personal level. The community of people living with HIV or AIDS is very varied. We are all very different people. We bring to our diagnoses a wide range of personal biographies, of understanding, of resources and of needs.

To build a 'community' of people with HIV or AIDS, with shared values, needs and objectives offering mutual support will be no easy task. We face enormous difficulties – stigma, isolation and fear. Above all, there are the difficulties of what has been described as 'living with uncertainty'. This is a daily constant in our lives.

The building of such an 'AIDS community' is helped by the courage of people living with HIV and AIDS and by their refusal to play a passive role. This in turn has been helped by their partnership with those voluntary agencies and professionals who have recognized the centrality of people with HIV and their perspective in their work.

All this takes place against a background of an increasing number of people with HIV and little prospect of a vaccine or cure. The need for greater public understanding – of the medical, social and personal effects – of the virus is paramount. This book will help promote that understanding.

Martyn Taylor
Chair, Board of Directors, Terrence Higgins Trust

SPONSOR'S FOREWORD

As the world's largest clothing maker, Levi Strauss & Co. has been involved in and committed to HIV/AIDS issues since 1982, when a group of employees asked for support from senior managers to help educate our people about a then new disease.

This was the beginning of our initiatives that now include employee education sessions; counselling and referral; grants and contributions to public education, patient care and AIDS agencies; involvement in development of sound public policy; and support for employee volunteer and fundraising efforts.

Education is the key. Education can build and change attitudes. It can help prevent the spread of HIV. It can alleviate ignorance that creates problems in workplaces, schools and communities.

That is why we continue to urge community, political and business leaders to make HIV/AIDS education a top priority – and a personal commitment.

I fervently hope this book serves as a contribution to the all-important education effort.

Robert D. Haas
Chairman and Chief Executive Officer
Levi Strauss & Co.

NOTES ON CONTRIBUTORS

The Terrence Higgins Trust is Europe's largest AIDS charity (and the second largest in the world), providing a range of services, advice and information to anyone affected by AIDS and HIV. Terrence Higgins died with AIDS in 1982. He was one of the first people to be diagnosed with AIDS in the United Kingdom and experienced intolerance, confusion and discrimination. His friends, shocked and saddened by the lack of information and support available, founded The Terrence Higgins Trust. Since 1983, 7,400 people have developed AIDS in the UK, of whom 4,600 have died. An estimated 30,000 people are thought to be infected with HIV, the virus that can lead to AIDS.

Network Photographers is one of Britain's foremost agencies for documentary photography. Since its foundation in 1981, the group's dedication to the coverage of serious issues at home and abroad has established Network as a leading exponent of intelligent reportage. Network Photographers publish internationally in books, magazines and newspapers, and are widely respected for editorial commitment and visual creativity.

Matt French is Gay Men's Health Officer at The Terrence Higgins Trust.

Eva Hayman is a Sister of the Society of the Holy Child Jesus and co-ordinator of the Family Network at The Terrence Higgins Trust.

Michael Mason is publisher of *Capital Gay*.

Pas Paschali is editor of *Him*.

ACKNOWLEDGEMENTS

This book and the related exhibition would never have been possible without the extraordinary commitment, generosity and courage of those affected by HIV and AIDS. We have been both inspired and moved by their experiences and have learnt so much from our collaboration with them.

The support and enthusiasm of Levi Strauss & Co. have been a constant source of strength during this challenging project. Their clear understanding of the issue and their humanity have been a vital part of this work. We are most grateful to them.

At the end of our first decade this exhibition and book reflect the Trust's uncompromising dedication to communicating the issues and human stories that arise from HIV and AIDS. We have had exceptional help from our colleagues, from the volunteers at The Terrence Higgins Trust and from others contributing to this project, including Holloway Prison and the Middlesex Hospital.

The photographers showed very special skills and sensitivity, and indeed we believe that the results are a glowing tribute to the founding principles of Network Photographers.

Our special thanks are due to Lynn O'Donoghue, Peter Ride, Claire Coulson, Barry Morse and Bryan McGregor of The Terrence Higgins Trust, all of whom made exceptional contributions to the realization of this project.

Stephen Mayes
Lyndall Stein

INTRODUCTION

PHOTOGRAPHING THE INVISIBLE –
A STATEMENT OF INTENT

There is something different about HIV and AIDS. If the photographers' purpose had been to explore the personal catastrophe of illness, there are many medical conditions that could have been approached. But, unlike any other virus, the medical and emotional battles of those living with HIV are underscored by unique social conditions. What distinguishes HIV and AIDS is not the illness, but the social and political context that has developed around it (it is hard to imagine any other medical condition that still receives more treatment in newsprint than in direct services to those affected). This work attempts to reflect some of these responses to the Human Immunodeficiency Virus.

These photographs show how the whole of society is involved with HIV: its transmission, the provision of care, the support structures, the attitudes and (when the virus strikes closer to home) the emotions. A medical condition has become a social condition, and we are all required to form a response and to accept a responsibility – whether by action, thought, or by simply trying to understand.

It is difficult to photograph illness in any meaningful way: pictures of people who are ill reveal very little beyond the physical symptoms of an invisible microbe's presence. But photography is extremely good at recording social conditions and offering interpretations of human experience. As with illness, many of the core subjects photographed here are invisible (feelings of love, fear, courage and alienation are no more visible than the physiological processes of a virus), but the process of photography translates these intangible miasmas into a recognizable form. Documentary photography has a power to communicate with an emotional immediacy that cannot be matched by words alone. This is greater than a mere descriptive exercise, for while these pictures use actuality as the raw material, the perceptions of the photographer and of the viewer stretch far beyond what is actually seen. With imagination as the added ingredient, these pictures put the viewer face to face with realities far beyond one's first-hand experience.

Positive Lives was conceived as a documentary project, and the photographers were selected for their ability to communicate rather than their previous exposure to the issues photographed. The function of documentary is to provide a record and, while journalistic integrity has been maintained throughout, subjective interpretation is an integral and equal part of such photography. Layered around this, the social climate that surrounds (and even shapes) the epidemic at the time of working imposes a political hue on the resulting body of work. Far from being a distraction, this adds depth to the project. From the outset it has been the intention to take stock of the wider social circumstances as we enter the second decade of AIDS care work in Europe, an opportunity to acknowledge truths that have been overlooked, many of which may still be considered distasteful. For while HIV and AIDS have obsessed the media to an enormous extent, many of the realities have been side-stepped, and these realities include the political as well as the medical and the emotional.

This work, which is presented as a book and as an exhibition, has two important contexts. The first is the present interpretation that viewers will read into the project and the lives of those photographed. Inevitably, there will be a huge diversity of responses – probably as many reactions to the work as there are to the illness itself: some will react with relief that their long-held secret feelings have been acknowledged; others will be angered by clashes of political belief; some will be shocked by confrontation with unimagined circumstances; many will be frustrated by the omission of significant realities. It is unlikely that any single viewer will identify with (or even recognize) all the experiences recorded here, but everyone who has a heart will be moved and it is to be hoped that many will also be strengthened by new knowledge to face the havoc that HIV will continue to wreak.

The second important context for this work will be future reference. At the time of production this book serves as a record of current experience, but in retrospect this will expand to offer a mirror reflecting a wider picture. This will not only provide information about a particular stage in the history of an epidemic, but will also serve as a record of social values and attitudes from far beyond the confines of 'planet AIDS' (as one commentator describes the beleaguered condition of those currently directly affected by HIV). By collating the skills and perspectives of several photographers working across a disparate range of subject matters and focusing on this single phenomenon, a coherent piece of social history emerges.

This project in itself is only part of the wider process of a society coming to terms with an illness and the particular issues that this illness has brought to the surface. No project dealing with these issues could hope to be comprehensive. AIDS is pandemic and the most obvious limitation on the scope of this project is geographic: all of this work was created within the British Isles. While this is a deliberate strategy to keep the project within manageable proportions and to keep attention concentrated on cultures and phenomena familiar to the participants, an attempt has been made to present as wide a range of responses as possible. Across these disparities and gaps, there is a coherent thread binding this work together: the shared experience of those directly affected by HIV in an uncomprehending society.

These are all real people and real lives. Their courage in identifying so closely with the problems that accompany HIV should not be underestimated in a culture that actively discriminates against people associated with this virus. By agreeing to be photographed, they are making a significant contribution to the understanding of an issue with which we are all involved. These are Positive Lives.

Stephen Mayes
Managing Editor, Network Photographers

CHAPTER 1

RESPONSES TO HIV

Photographs by Denis Doran

HIV and AIDS affect everyone. The people in these photographs are not necessarily HIV-positive.

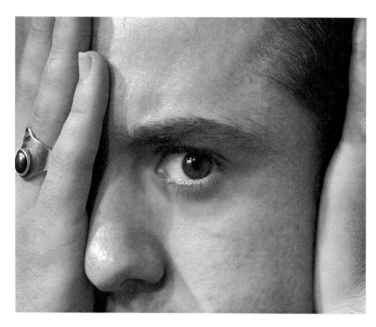

'Why should I be made to feel isolated amongst the people I live with?' *Murad*

'So you think it's just *their* problem?' *Julian*

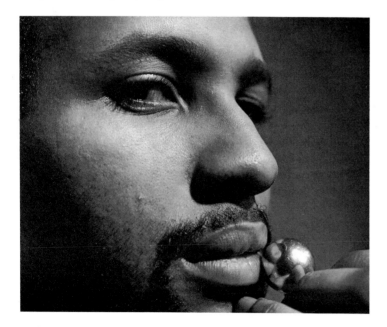

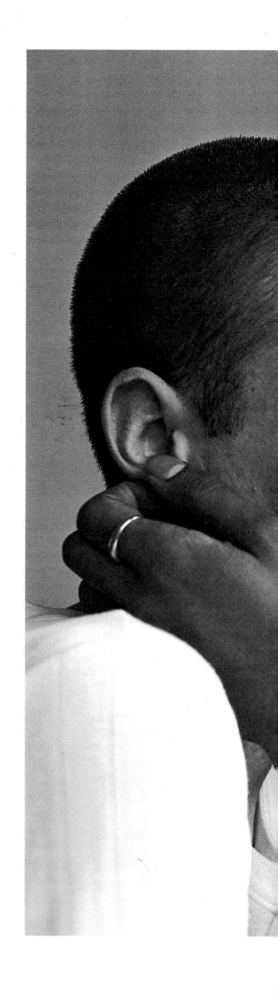

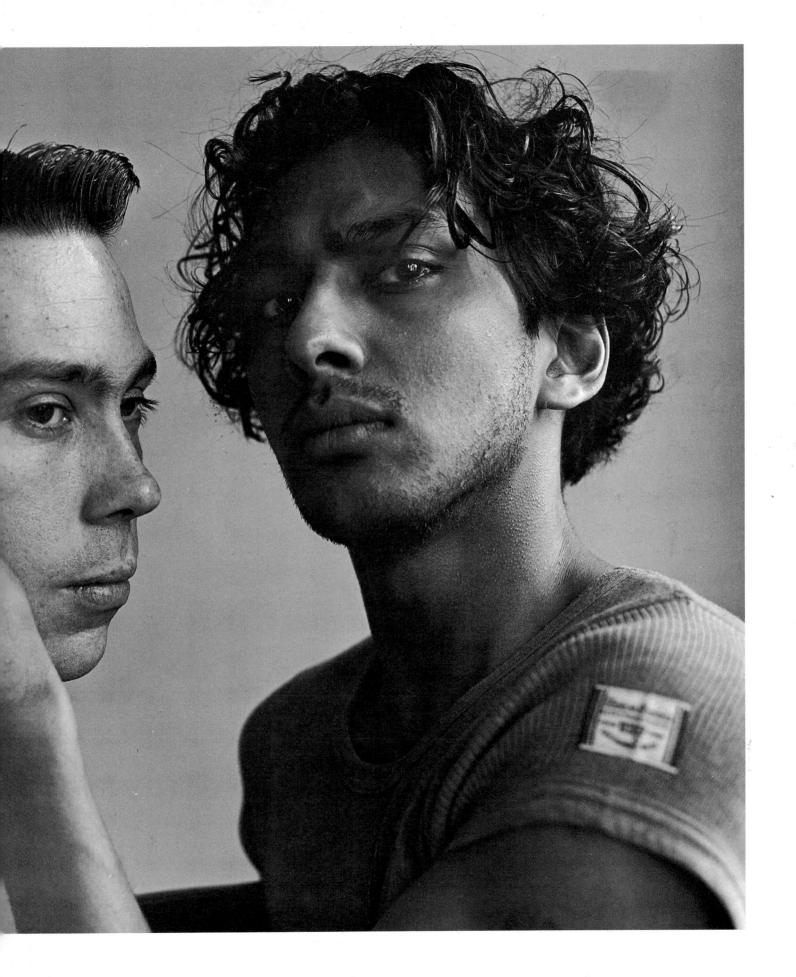

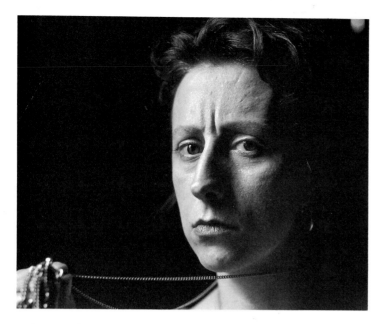

'What? I will not stay silent.' *Mary Jane*

'Just what are *you* doing?' *Filiz*

'The irrational fear of homosexuality stifles man's ability to love.
Whatever his sexuality, my son must learn to open himself to love
those around him.' *Gill and Jake*

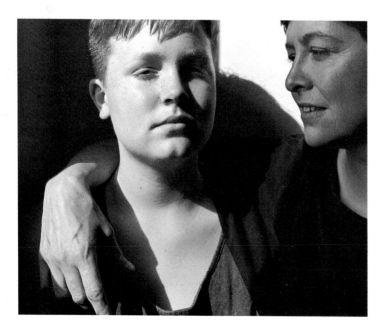

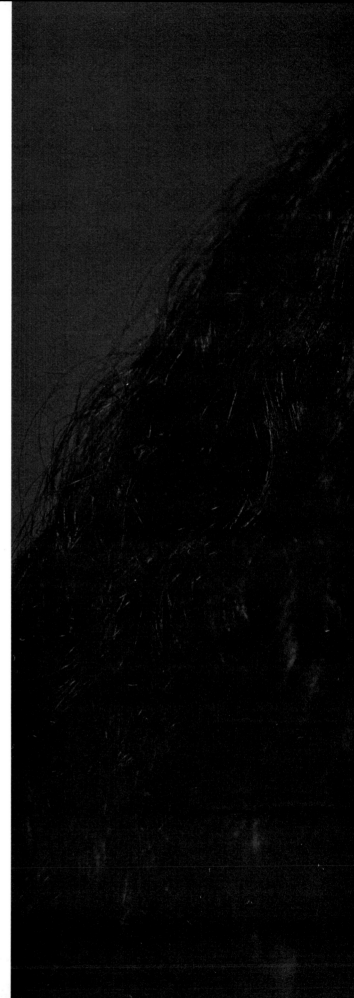

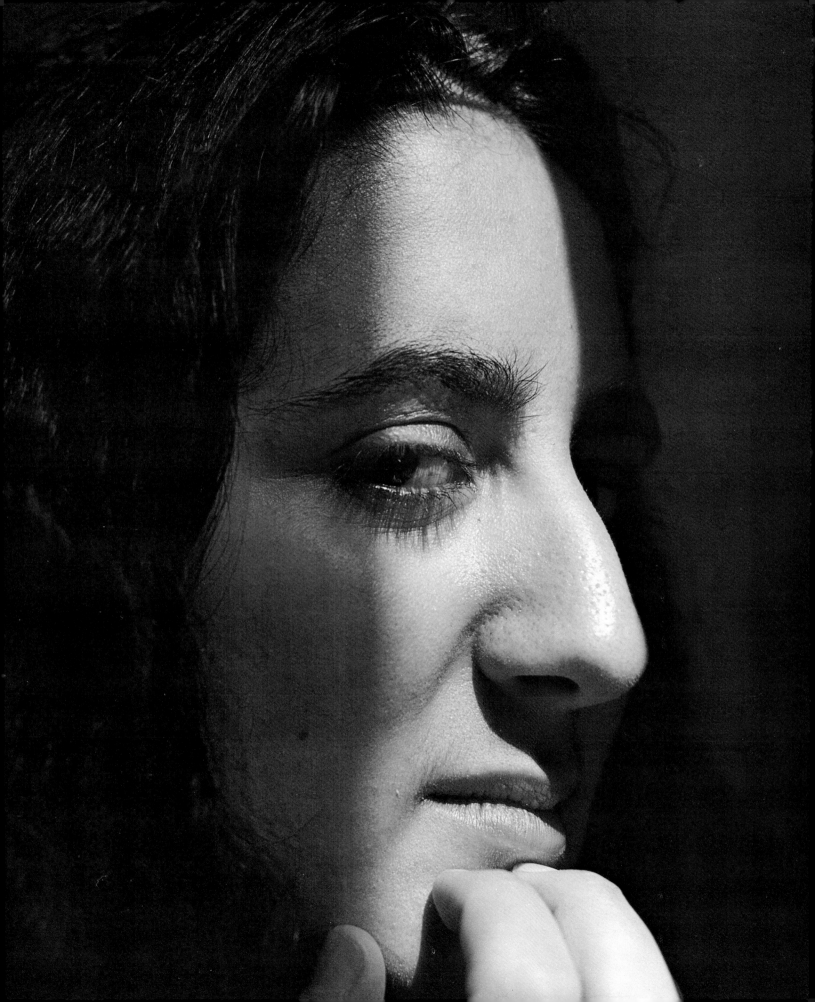

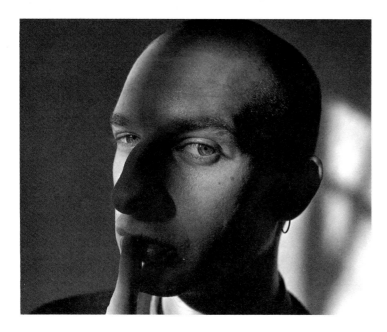

'Silence = death.' *Ian*

'It's possible that sooner or later we'll all know someone who's positive.' *Olly*

'As lesbians we smile at general ignorance.' *Sharlie*

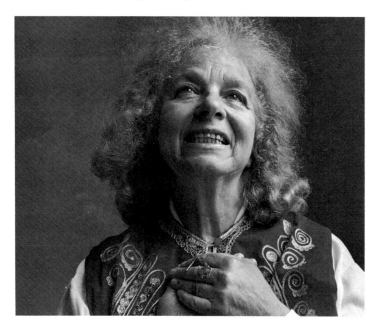

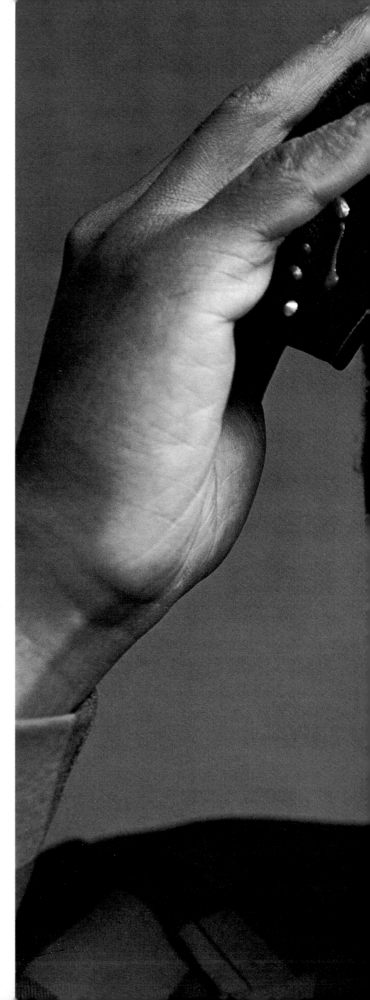

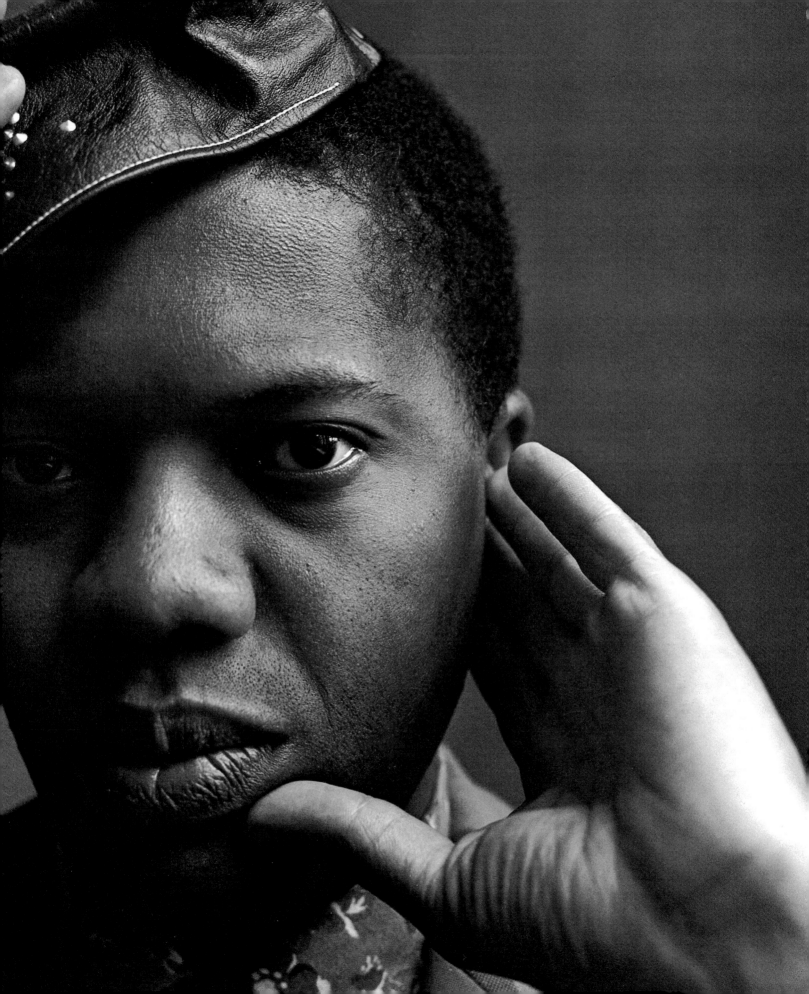

CHAPTER 2

THE ESTATE – A Family Secret

Photographs by John Sturrock

In 1987 the work of Roy Robertson, an Edinburgh doctor working with young drug users at the Muirhouse Housing Estate, attracted the attention of television and newspapers. He had discovered that many of the users were HIV-positive and some had already developed AIDS. In January 1988, photographer John Sturrock made his first trip to the estate and started a relationship with the place and some of its inhabitants.

'Tragic issues – war, crime, deprivation – usually provide the subject matter for photojournalism. The pictures are rarely about the issue. They are about victims, and they often describe threats to the fundamental needs of human survival.

'Yet we have other needs, emotional, often unconscious, and just as important for our well-being. If we ignore these needs and the subsequent symptoms, in the way we keep a "family secret", then, as with all such secrets, what is not recognized is incomprehensible.

'In Muirhouse I witnessed the emotional struggle of people enduring a tragedy. I also began to notice moments of love and intimacy. They were the clues, which sometimes I was able to photograph. A framework is necessary in order to help us assimilate these clues.

'In the sixties the photographs from the Vietnam war were shocking, but there was a purpose, a way of receiving them: the protest movement at the time.

'However, there is no external context to help us rationalize photographs of self-abuse. We have to look inside ourselves, to our own patterns of need and denial, and having touched our own pain, we might be generous about that of others.'

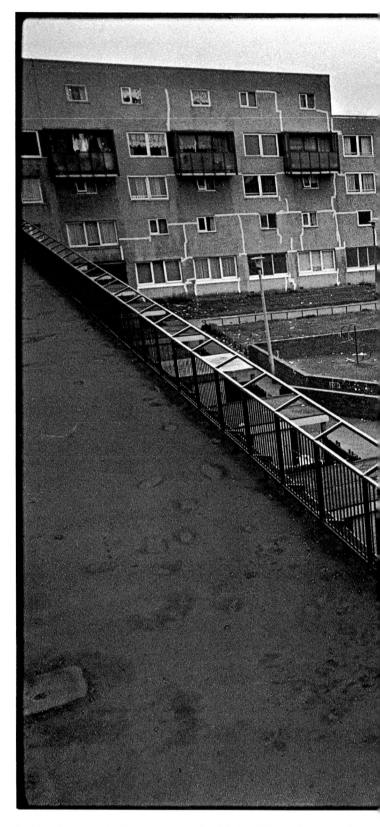

In this grim system-built environment, devoid of facilities and jobs, people find it almost impossible to connect with the familiar, thriving, healthy and well-resourced face of Edinburgh.

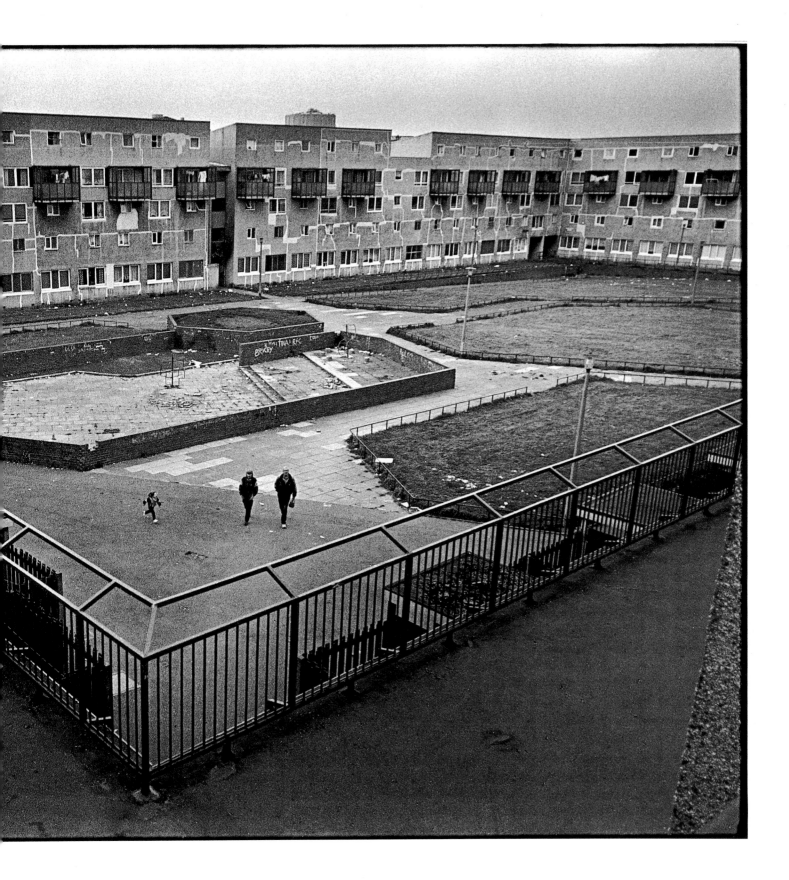

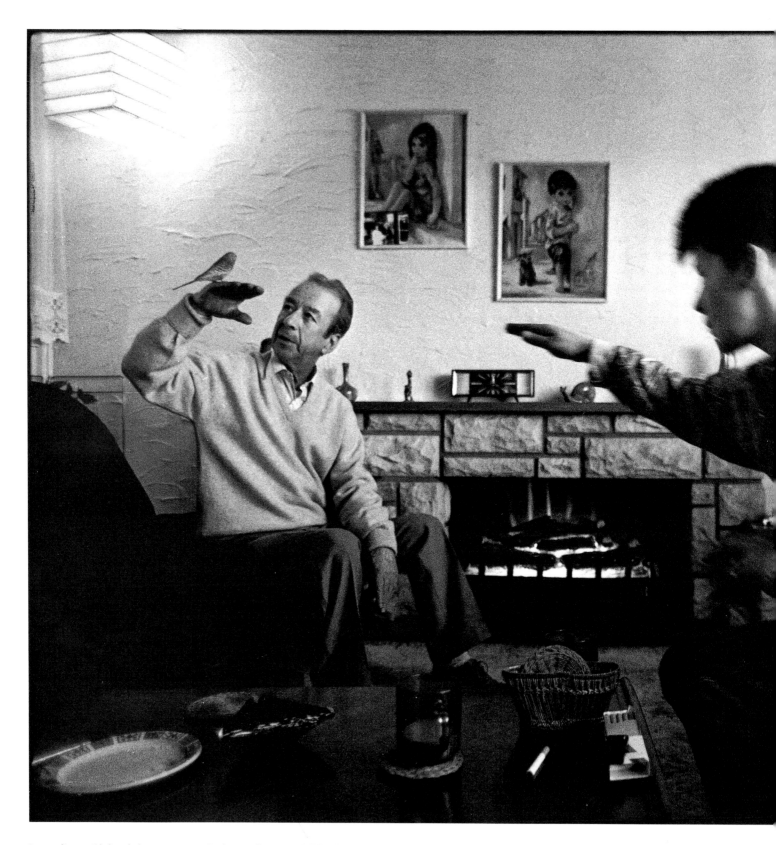

Lynne lives with her father, Joe. He retired at 59, because of ill health, and he misses his work. His wife died 12 years ago, while Lynne was in prison. She was heavily into drugs when she was released. She was diagnosed HIV-positive in 1984. Lynne and Joe look after each other. The budgie, Timmy, was a present which she gave him on his fifty-ninth birthday.

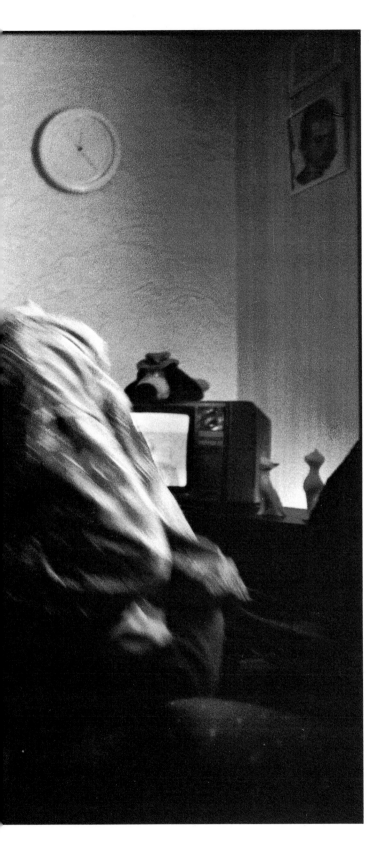

LYNNE

On her wall there is a poster. She has carefully filled in the blank spaces. It reads:

PRISONER: LYNNE HALEY; PRISON NUMBER 163/89; SENTENCE: LIFE

Eventually her niece Tippexed out LIFE.

Lynne is renowned for her exploits. She describes what happened to her in 1989.

'I heard the police coming into the block of flats, and I knew they were after me. I was on the first floor in the corridor above the shops. There was no other exit, so I ran through an open front door, past the family watching TV, and jumped out of a window.

'I smashed both my ankles. A friend found me. He ripped open the legs of my jeans because of the swelling, carried me into the back of a nearby shop, and called an ambulance. They gave me laughing gas as a pain killer. It was so good that I asked them to take the long way round to the hospital.

'I reckoned that the police would find me in the hospital, so my boyfriend helped me escape. He was pushing me down the corridor in a wheelchair, when a doctor tried to stop us by grabbing hold of it, so my boyfriend carried me out on his back. We went straight to the pub for double vodkas. I was wearing great big sponge shoes and the ripped jeans.

'It was four or five months before they caught me shoplifting on crutches. I was bailed because I was due to have an operation on my ankles. I was caught twice more before they refused bail. Three months later, my ankles were sorted out.'

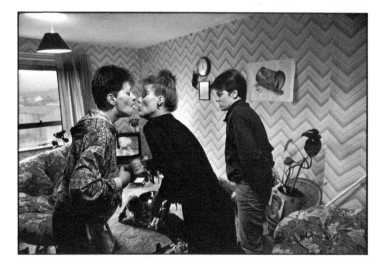

Lynne, Trisha and Donna in Trisha's flat.

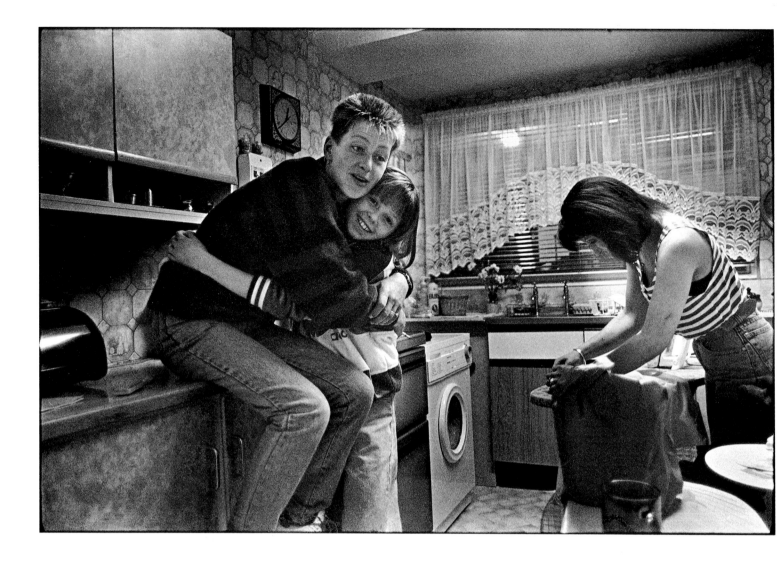

Lynne, on the night before she goes to a drug rehabilitation centre, with her niece, Kerry. Her sister irons clothes for the trip.

Joe and Timmy wait for Lynne's return from the drug rehabilitation centre. She only stayed there one night, and then disappeared for a few days. Joe reported her missing to the police, but they said that there was little they could do as she was over sixteen. When she returned to Edinburgh, she explained that she had left because she felt that it was worse than being in prison.

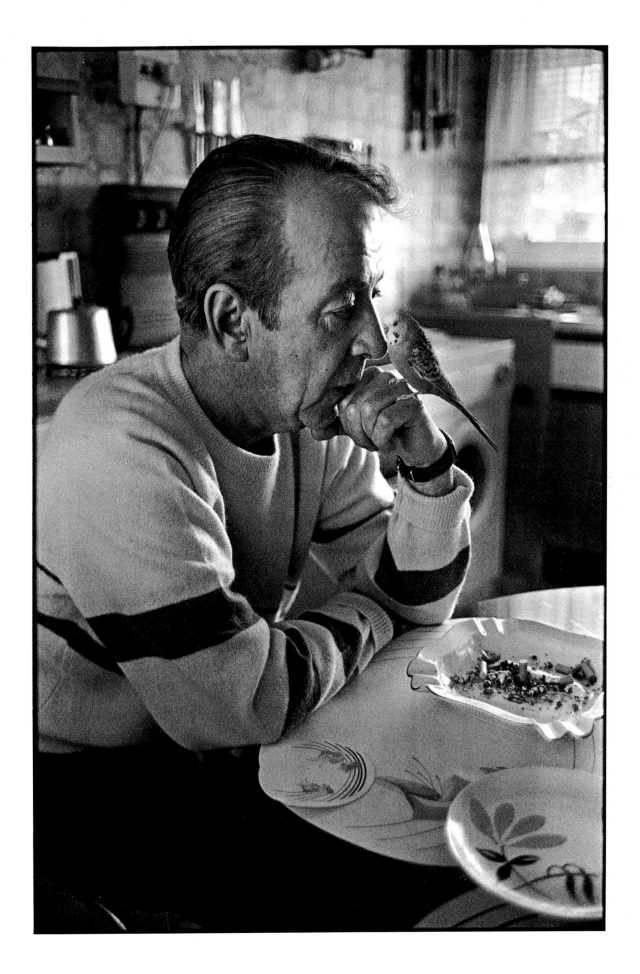

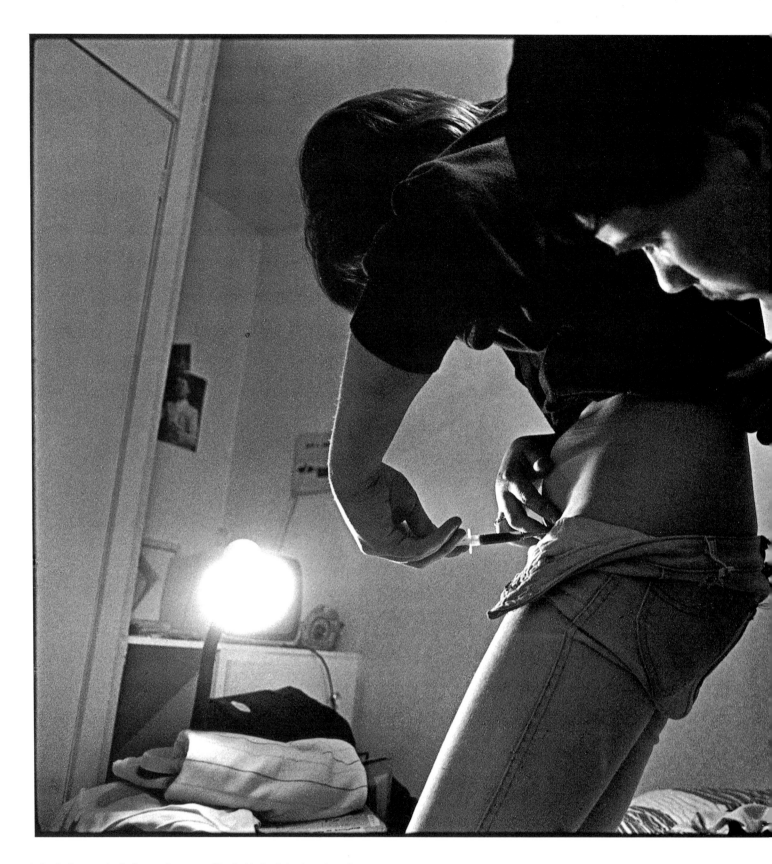

Only the large veins in her groin were still suitable for injecting; the others had hardened from use. It is a dangerous practice, and they helped each other get a 'hit'. On this occasion, there was a problem with the needle, and he was concerned for her.

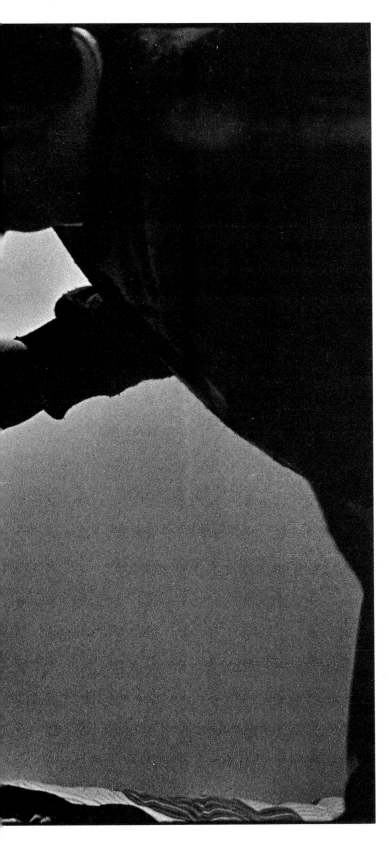

THE HIT

'Les! Les!'

The big lad's shout was heartfelt. He bangs on the door. Inside we go quiet and I shrink into my chair. I've seen him before in his thick white jumper, jeans and brogues. And his pain. I don't know whether to fear or hug him. His emotions are displayed like entrails. They are all like that. Wasted bodies, childish behaviour, crushing me. I absorb it, like punishment, knowing that later it will haunt me.

He bangs on the door. She curses quietly and tells him to go away, she's trying to sleep, she'll see him later. He sighs and leaves us.

I know when I meet him next he will have heard that they had taken me to her room so that I could watch and photograph, and he had been excluded. He'll know that I saw the woman he wanted in her underclothes – hunched over, slowly puncturing her groin with a needle – with her companion, naked and triumphant, calling over to me, his blood-filled syringe hanging beside his penis.

When I left them – in their cotton-wool, clogged euphoria – I stroked her face, telling her to take care. I felt stupid. And when the door closed behind me, I felt cold and hard, like the concrete buildings.

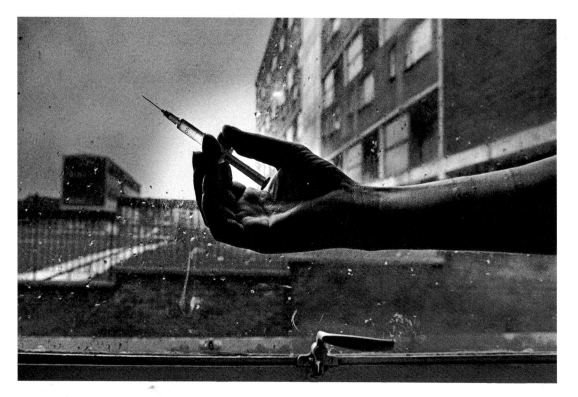

Graham's flat.

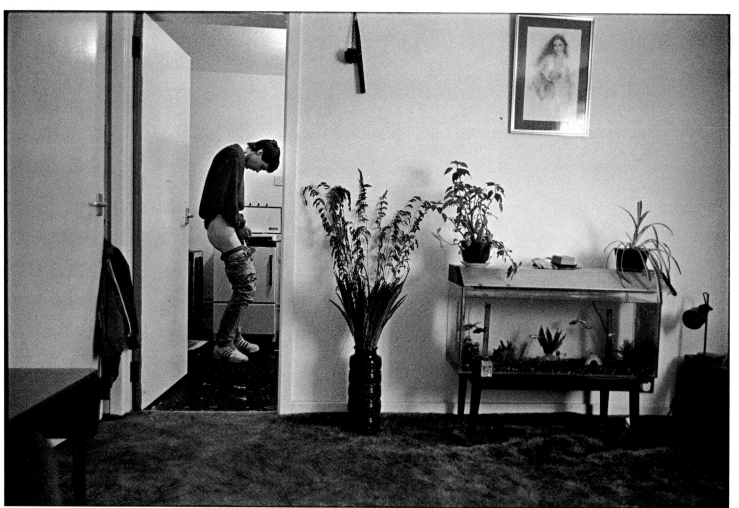

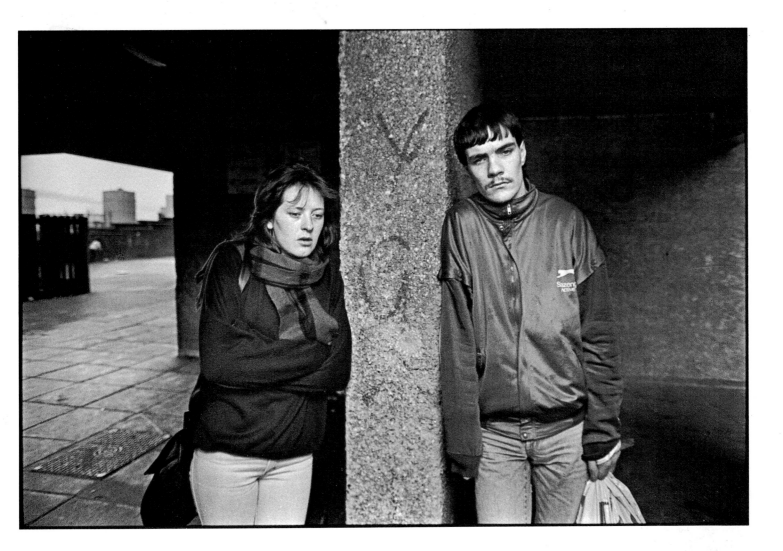

A bus trip into the city for a meeting with Graham's solicitor.

Graham is reunited with a friend who has just been released from prison.

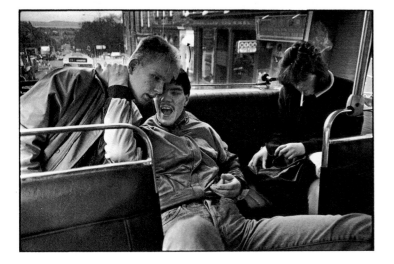

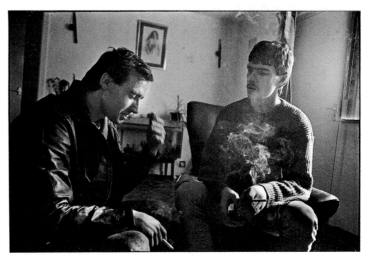

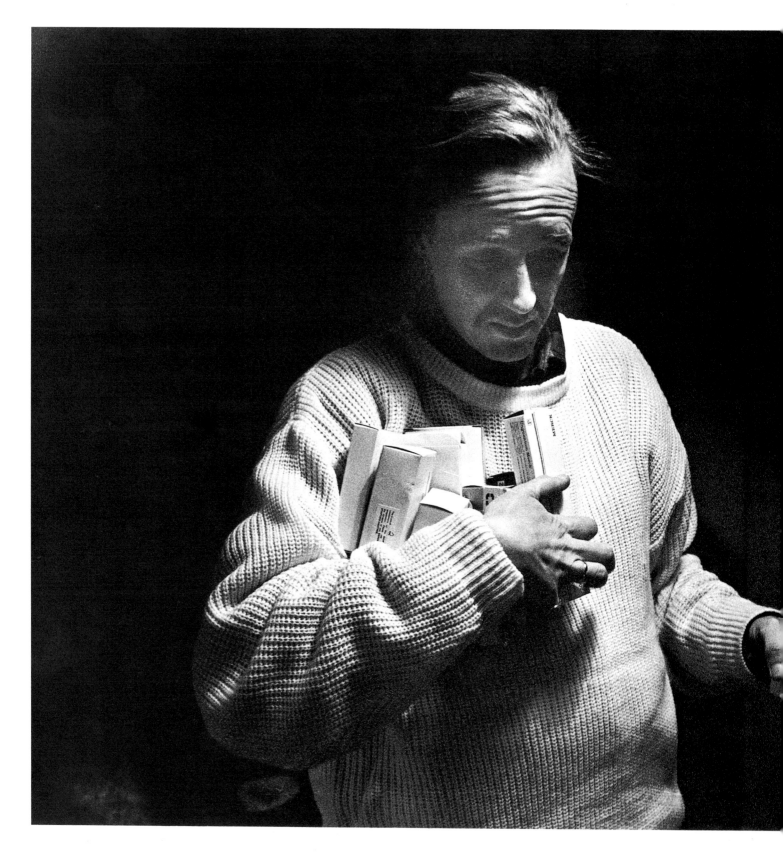

In one arm, Vince carries his daily medication for his symptoms; in the
other, the antidotes for the side-effects.

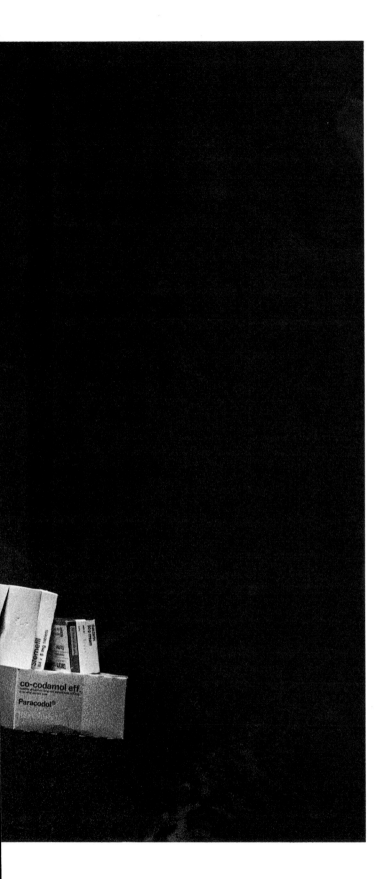

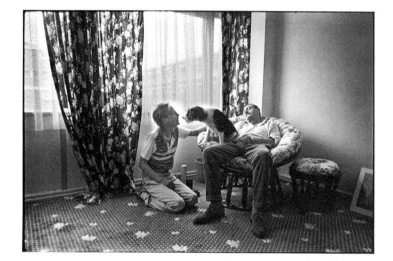

Vince and Hugh lived together as a couple. After Vince was diagnosed as HIV-positive in November 1989, Hugh gave up work to look after him.

In 1984 Vince worked for a time as a rent boy in London. Two years later he returned to Edinburgh, working as a male stripper, then as a super-market assistant. His last job was radio controller for a taxi firm. He died in 1992.

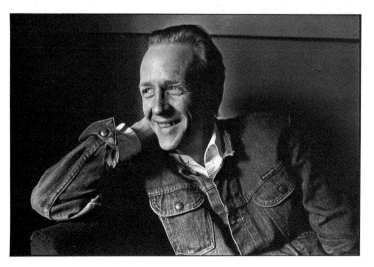

TRISHA

It's a year since I last faced the wind that swirls around the tower block. The entryphone warbles and eventually she answers. This time I am recognized and invited up, but either she forgot or there's a fault; the door won't open.

Shadows move behind the armoured glass. Two narrow-faced youths emerge and eye me.

'All right mate?' They hold the heavy door open, and I escape inside.

The lift opens and I face the battered door to her flat. Her eyes are clear and a smile spreads more smoothly across her face than I remember.

'Hello Trisha. You're looking good.'

'Och, I don't feel it. I haven't even got my makeup on.'

The room is familiar, but slightly less chaotic. The same zig-zag striped wallpaper, the last drop still missing, but now hung with an airbrushed poster of a crumpled Coke can and the large plastic relief of a Santa head. The scars in the plaster have gone.

Simon comes in, as small and sweet as ever; he doesn't remember me, but he still has the photos. He lies down in front of the TV to watch a video. He's wearing a football shirt. I ask him which team.

'It's Hearts. Who do you support?'

'Dundee. My dad wanted to play for them.'

He feigns laughter and digs into a packet of crackers. Carefully he spreads marge onto one of them.

She is watching him and pulling faces.

'I've told you to be careful, and no more after this one.'

He grins at me, puts his hand in the pocket and pulls out another.

'Simon', her voice is suddenly brittle and exasperated. 'I told you, no more.'

He takes a bite.

'Well, no more after this, you wee monkey.'

The anger fades and her face relaxes.

'You should have seen it here at Christmas, everything was maroon and white. Hats, scarves, football strip – even clocks.'

He looks up at her sharply.

'I know, clocks that don't work,' she says wearily.

'We'll get the money back.'

Momentarily she is silent, staring at the floor.

'Where are your football boots?'

He mumbles a reply.

'At Granma's,' she exclaims with renewed exasperation. 'But she's gone away for two months, aye, in Australia for two months, sunning herself. Still she deserves it after her life', she continues for my benefit.

'She's not gone yet, not till the eighteenth.'

Trisha's face folds in confusion. 'She went on the first, didn't she?'

'No she didn't.' He looks at me, rolls his eyes and waggles a finger towards the side of his head.

Head bowed and muttering, she repeats the arguments to herself.

'Simon got football mad at his Granma's. He was there for three months while I was in hospital. Three months they had me – it sounds like prison,' she chuckles. 'I had pneumonia. I had to have oxygen. I had the choice of a mask or tubes.'

Now I'm confused.

'You know, up my nostrils.' She demonstrates with two thin fingers.

The sound of guns firing on the video catches and holds our attention. Errol Flynn ducks and runs.

'The box said it was *Paint Your Wagon*, but we got this.'

A bar-room brawl breaks out, pandemonium, cowboys fighting, tables and chairs flying and bodies falling from balconies.

Simon rubs his hands with glee, and says, 'Ah, Muirhouse!'

He looks at me, puts a finger to his lips and dips his other hand into the cracker box.

'That's enough, I've told you.' A harsh strength grates in her voice. He looks up at me like a scolded puppy, resting his cheek on his knee.

He stacks cracker box and marge on the plate and carries them with both hands to the kitchen. At the door he crouches and turns the handle with his mouth.

'Why's he not at school?'

She says something about his broken tooth, but then admits she has been sleeping from 9.30 in the evening until midday.

'Last Saturday you slept till seven in the evening,' he says, reappearing from the kitchen. I hear her echo his words.

'The doctor says I'm not fully recovered from my illness, and he's cut back on my pills. I'm trying, but if somebody is selling, I'll buy a fiver's worth. That's why I stay in most of the time, so I won't be tempted. It's such a trap. I've got to get the hell out of here. I've got to give the wee fella a chance. When they gave me my backdated money, I left him a trust.'

I look round to see if Simon is listening, but there's no sign of him.

I stand up, I must leave soon. I look down at her. I see thin legs wrapped around each other, reminiscent of high heels and bar stools.

Sometimes, because of her symptoms and the effects of the medicine, Trisha finds it hard to wake up in the morning.

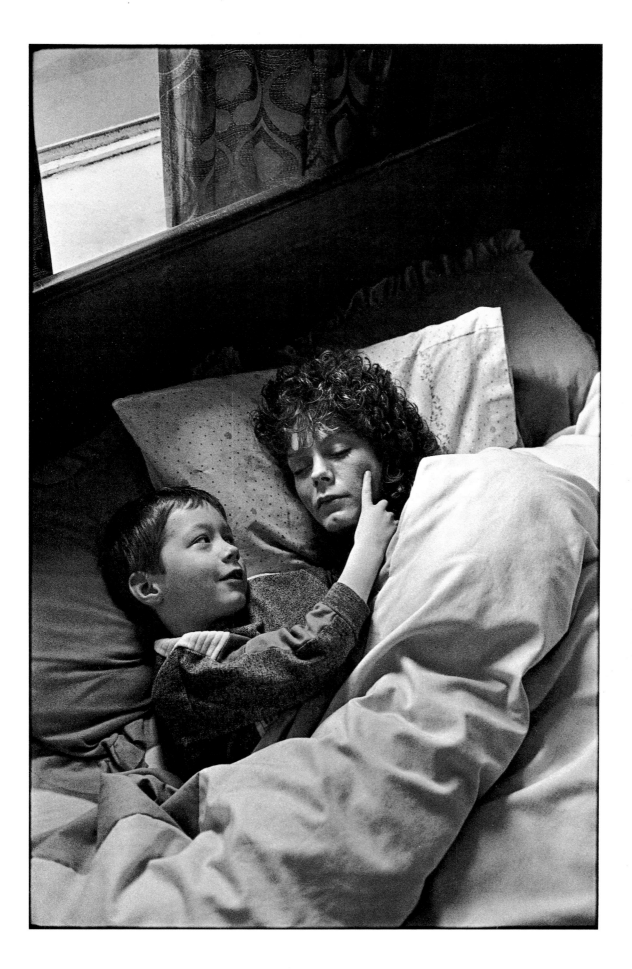

35

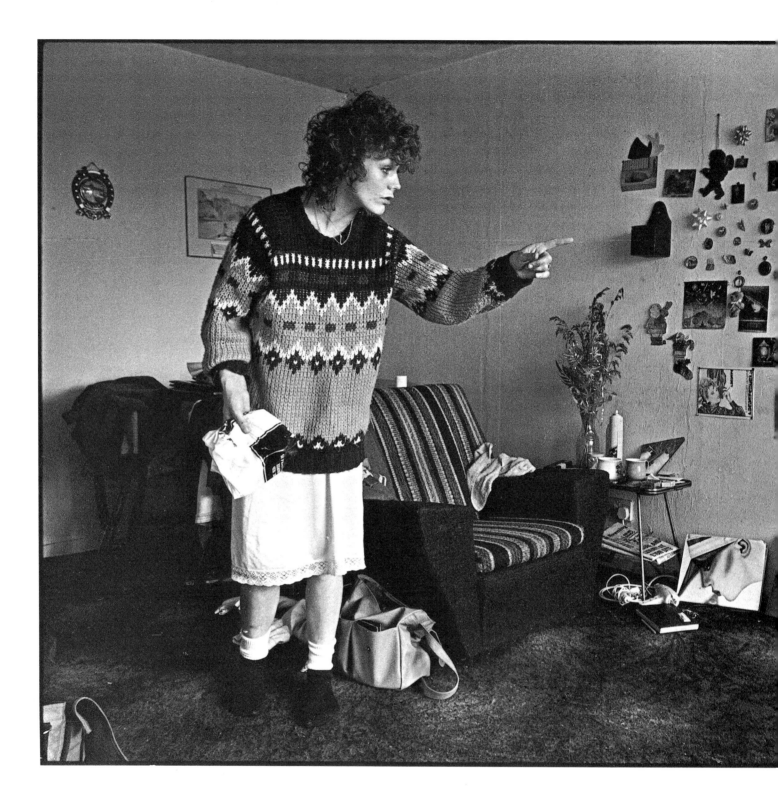

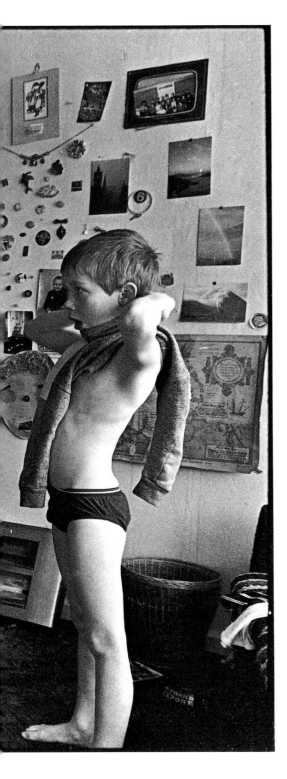

As we walk through the hallway, I look into her bedroom, and see the duvet moving on her bed. Simon is hiding beneath it. I call to him to come and say goodbye, but he just replies with a muffled 'Bye'.

'You must see his Christmas present,' she says, opening the door to his bedroom. In amongst the clashing colours and torn wall-paper, I make out a smart grey combined platform bed and desk and a matching set of drawers.

'We got it from the showroom, into the van, through the front door, but it wouldn't fit in the lift. We had to take it apart down there, in the lobby, and bring it up bit by bit.'

I wonder if Simon will come to take possession of his room, and show off his present, but he remains silent in his mother's bed.

We return to the hall and she opens the front door.

She holds out her hand for a formal goodbye. I hold onto it, and she leans forwards to kiss me.

'Remember, the door's always open,' she calls as I walk down the stairwell.

John Sturrock

Trisha appeared on a TV programme, admitting that even though she knew she was HIV-positive, she continued to work as a prostitute. There was resentment and open hostility towards her and her son. She felt that many people were hypocritical.

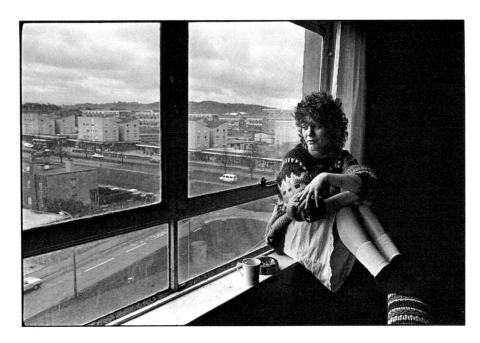

CHAPTER 3

PRISON

Photographs by Michael Abrahams

HIV and AIDS are locked away with the prisoners of every such institution, adding pressures to already pressurized lives.

In 1988 the Home Office estimated that 0.1% of inmates in British jails were HIV-positive. However, at the same time, studies in Europe revealed that in Switzerland the figure was 11%, in France 12.6%, in the Netherlands 11% and in Spain 18.7%. It is reasonable to suppose that out of our prison population of 50,000, some 8,000 people are carrying the virus.

The Government has been spending millions of pounds on a publicity campaign to drive home warnings of the dangers of AIDS and the importance of safe sex. It has given the go-ahead for needle exchange schemes to be set up around the country. Research suggests that 6% of all male, and 16% of all female, prisoners were drug offenders.

In prison culture, needles or syringes are reported to have a greater value than the drug itself because of their scarcity. The Government will not condone the illegal use of drugs in prison by operating a needle exchange.

HOLLOWAY

These pictures make no distinction between those who do and don't have the virus, allowing them to speak for themselves and the viewers to consider their prejudices and preconceptions. These pictures were made in Holloway, London's prison for women.

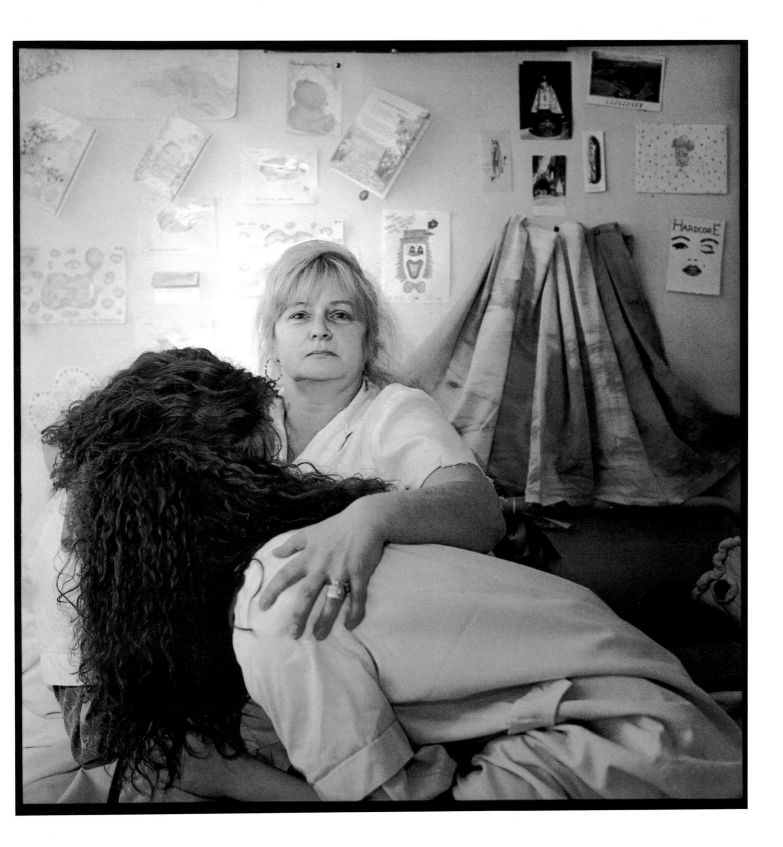

'We've all shared the room with her for months so why should she be taken away from us? When she was in the hospital, I took people with me to visit her to show her that people did care. If you have a bad cold, you don't want to go near them. You can kill them, they can't kill you.'

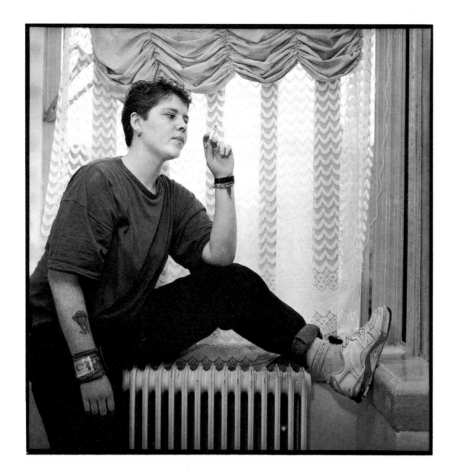

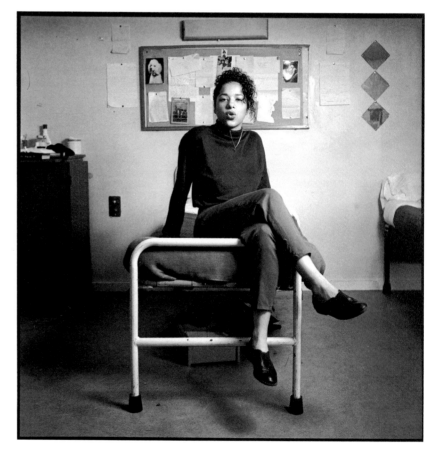

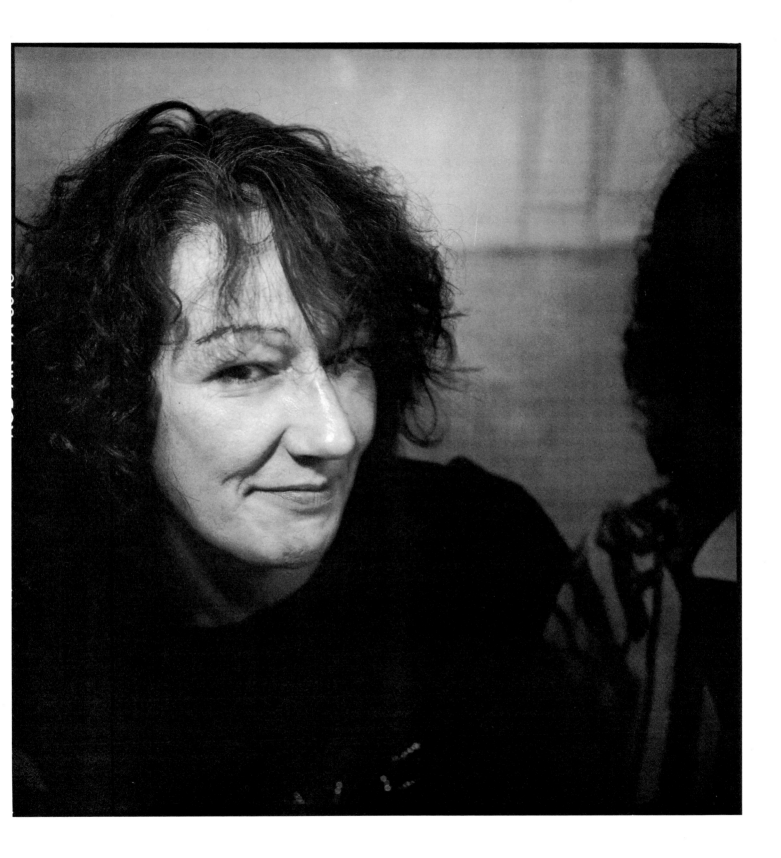

'Why should I have a test? I've got two and a half years to do; why risk
making it into a life sentence?'

THE MOUNT – Men's Prison

'I was diagnosed HIV-positive in 1985. I wasn't an intravenous drug user, I didn't have sex with men, I'd just recently left my wife and had picked up with another woman for about a year. I ignored the fact that I was positive and didn't even think about it – I just wasn't HIV-positive as far as I was concerned. After about two years I found myself in prison and I just couldn't get away from it. When I arrived at reception in the jail, the police told them that I was HIV-positive. As I didn't want to have another test – I don't like needles – I was put in a strip cell for four days. It was a really bad turning-point. I was isolated, I was getting fed through the door, I had no contact with anyone. My name on the notice board had big red flashes all over it; my folder in the office had yellow stickers on saying 'Danger – Contamination'. I was really depressed at being locked up anyway, and I was even more depressed because of the situation. I couldn't understand it; if I was this contagious I wouldn't have been on the street walking about. It was a ludicrous situation where I couldn't keep it quiet even if I'd wanted to.

'When I submitted to having the test again in prison, the number one inmate on the wing, not even the hospital wing, got a message to me to tell me that my test was positive. I had been to the doctor for my results and he'd said they weren't back yet. So I went to the Governor and he told me that they were in fact back and were in the doctor's office. So obviously the inmate had been in there and he came and told me the results of my HIV test. That's shit, that's real shit.

'So then I was put on the landing but I was isolated from the rest of the inmates. I wasn't allowed to go to the gym and I wasn't allowed to work.

'It was my local jail; I'd been going there on and off for about ten years. Most of the officers knew me. Out of 400 people there, about 150 knew my face and about 100 probably knew me. After about four months of people seeing me and mixing with me, and people knowing me for so long, the HIV sort of disappeared – they forgot about it. But you still got the diehards shouting down the landing. I didn't want to leave as it was OK after five months. I was near my home, my family, health care – the hospital was right across the road.

'I got shipped out to Dartmoor. Winchester didn't want an HIV prisoner any more. Dartmoor rejected me. Camp Hill rejected me. Normal blokes go to prison and the officers are there to keep them there, but those officers want people like me out. So the same night I was back at Winchester. They put me in a cell with no bed, nothing. So I kicked the door – got nicked and ended up down the block.

'Things were getting awkward there so I wrote to the Governor at Camp Hill. I said I've been no trouble, I'm going to get shipped miles away if you don't accept me. As I had a commendation, I could use it as a bargaining chip.

'When I arrived at Camp Hill I went onto the landing. It was a small wing of about thirty people, and they all knew someone was coming on with AIDS. I had a hard time. Officers wouldn't talk to me, they'd avoid me. The inmates were 98% Londoners and I didn't know anybody. During that time I really had to go over-board in making everyone feel safe with me. You couldn't share a joint, you'd never offer your cup to anyone. Sharing is so important to your relationships in prison.

'If I was in the shower, I couldn't say, "Give us a go of your soap." At Camp Hill I was in one house block for seven months, and it just started to become OK. Then I got nicked for wiring my radio up to the light. It's not such a serious offence; everyone's at it. So I was moved to a much bigger house block. Again I didn't know anyone and had to start all over again.

'Then I was moved to the Mount and had to start all over again. When I got there I was told that there was no need to disclose my HIV status: "Our policy is one of strict confidentiality." So I said, "All right, I'll do that." I thought it would be nice to be normal.

'After about four weeks someone from Camp Hill arrived. Then one dinner time someone says to me, "You've got AIDS."

'I said, "No, I'm HIV-positive."

'Then, "Fucking hell – we don't want you on this wing." So they stirred up a load of trouble, and we were all banged up, except for four who refused to be banged up. They spoke with the Prison Officer, and half an hour later I was the one down the block for four days.

'At least if you're a sex offender, you're with other sex offenders, you're all together. Being HIV-positive is worse than being a sex offender. The screws don't publicize the fact that you're a sex offender.'

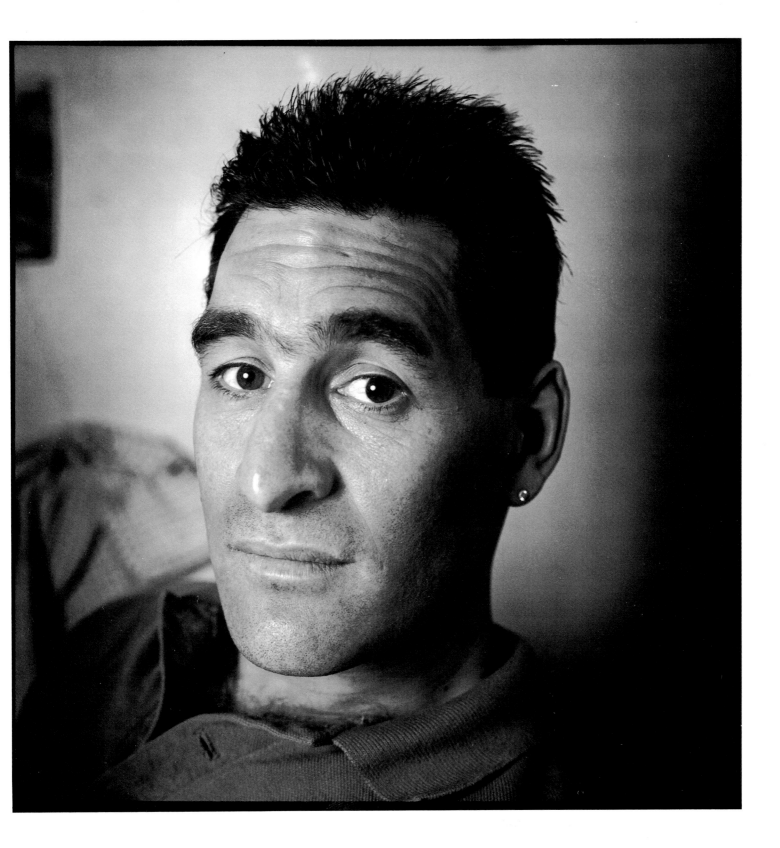

'I was diagnosed as being HIV-positive seven years ago. This is the most secure jail in Europe. You've seen the security – they're so paranoid. Two weeks ago I really slashed myself up and I needed 54 stitches. The last cut was really bad because I cut an artery and so lost a few pints of blood. I'm not suicidal, just self-destructive. When they see someone spouting blood they just freak. With anyone else they'd be jumping all over them, but they're just terrified of me. I just wind them up – that's what they're there for, it's better than anti-depressants.

'When they took me by ambulance to the hospital the place was full of people who'd been in accidents and that, and then there was me; I felt a bit ashamed because my injuries were self-inflicted. I decided I wasn't going to die easily. I was going to fight like fuck. It was a sort of turning-point in my life. I wasn't going to have them sitting in their mess just saying "So there's another one off". Now I'm really at peace with myself. It's the first time in my life that I've been pleased to wake up in the morning. This has taught me a good lesson which I wouldn't have missed for anything.

'I'm not doing two life sentences for shoplifting. I don't stand for any crap. I'm not scared of dying, there's nothing to be scared of. These places can do nothing and being locked up doesn't bother me but being in prison does.

'There are lots of prisons on the outside. Living in a cardboard box is a life sentence. I don't need to escape, like the way some need to with drugs. I could be rich in here, you can get £50 for a syringe, but I don't approve of drugs.

'I was a prostitute, a rent boy. I've never regretted anything – except the circumstances that got me in here; I live for now. Yesterday's the past. Tomorrow's a dream.'

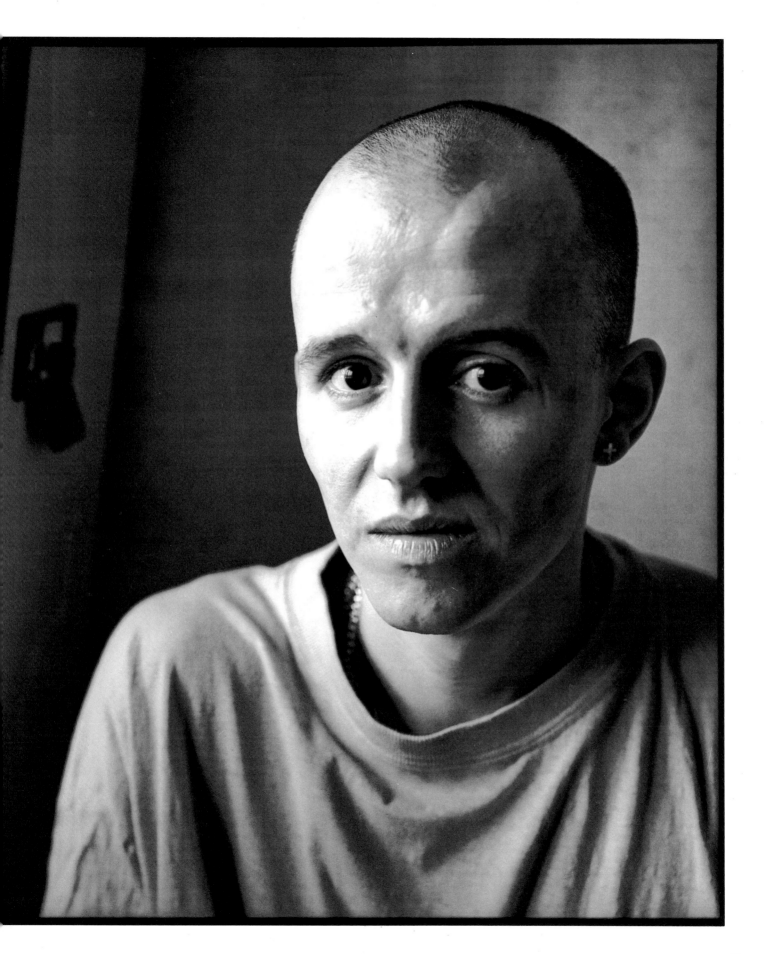

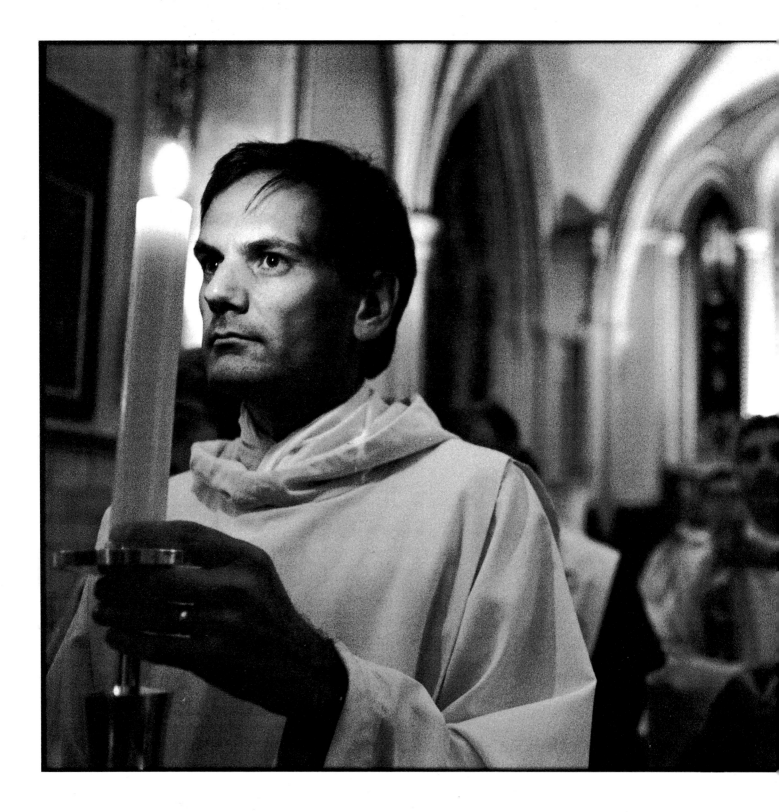

A priest, holding the AIDS Memorial Candle, leads the procession which begins a specially composed Requiem Mass at Southwark's Anglican Cathedral dedicated to those affected by HIV and AIDS. The Requiem, composed by Gareth Valentine, played to a full Cathedral.

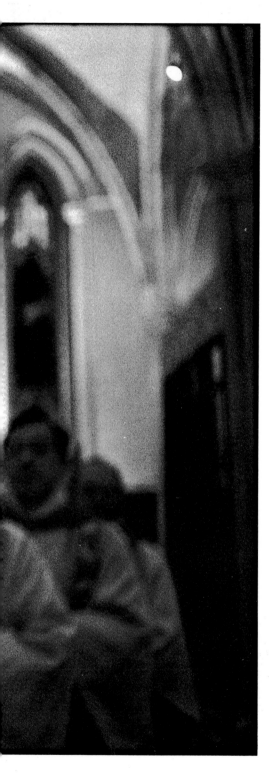

CHAPTER 4

RELIGIOUS RESPONSE –
The Body of Christ Has AIDS

Photographs by Mike Goldwater

Initially, church responses to HIV and AIDS were often fearful. It has taken time for this to change, and for a more appropriate response to replace prejudice and lack of understanding. Paradoxically, the very people who were often stigmatized and rejected have enabled individual Christians and church communities to become more compassionate.

Through ignorance, people with HIV and AIDS are often regarded as 'them' – not one of us. However, as Christians from many different churches are combining to meet the needs of people with HIV and AIDS, they are discovering that brokenness is part of our common humanity and not the lot of one stigmatized group.

No one person or organization can meet all the needs of another. The challenge of AIDS is enabling individuals and Church groups to combine their resources, to open their doors and their hearts and to work together to meet the spiritual and pastoral needs of people with AIDS, their partners, families and carers. This calls for a non-judgemental inclusive response and there are many signs that this is beginning to happen.

The next step will be to allow the ecumenical response to develop into an interfaith movement and to recognize within this the part played by the unchurched, that large number of committed believers who have been rejected by various religious institutions.

When this develops, AIDS will be seen and experienced as All In the Divine Service.

Eva Hayman

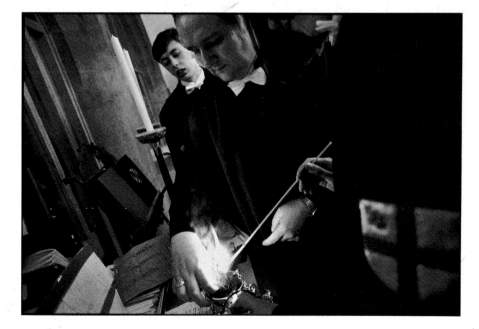

Lighting incense before the beginning of the Requiem Mass. Southwark Cathedral was the first church in Britain to dedicate a chapel to those affected by HIV and AIDS.

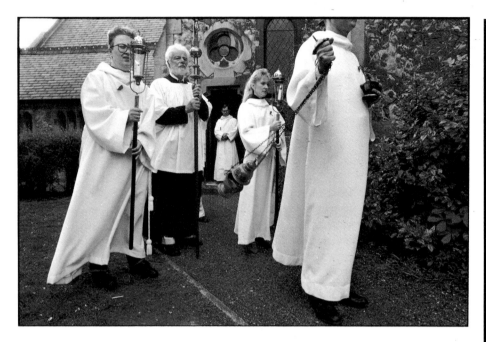

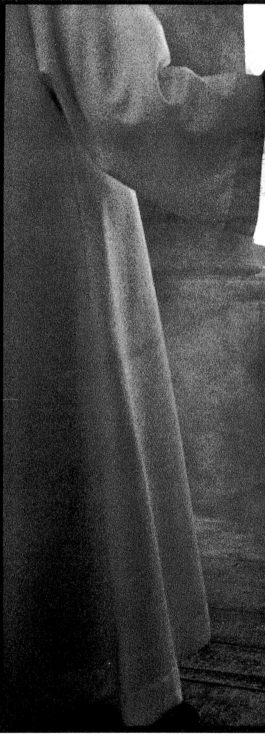

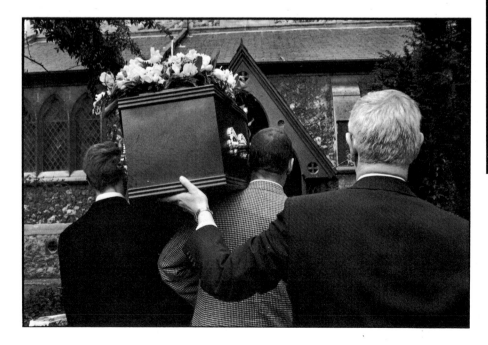

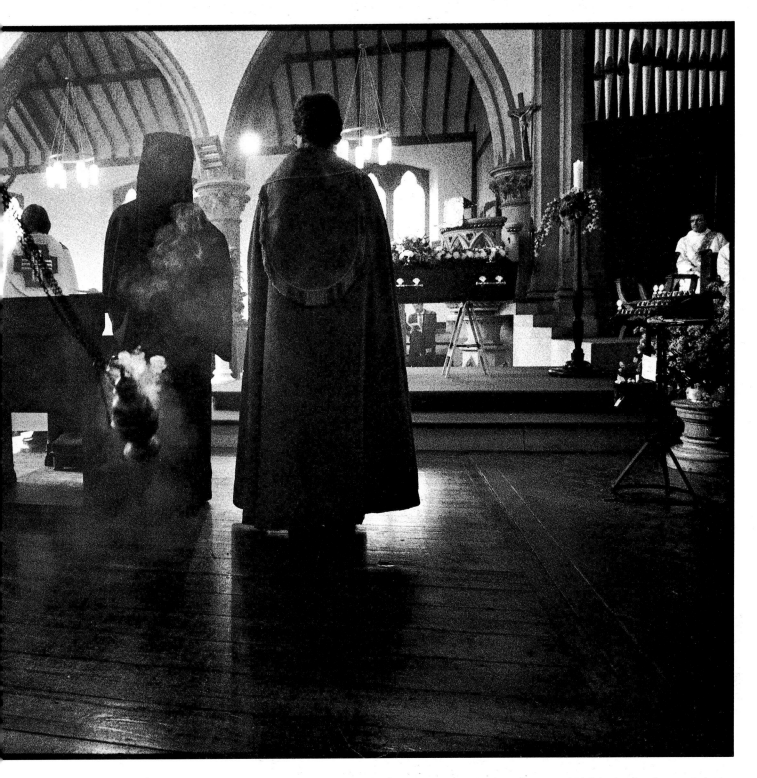

Charalambos Sophianos, 36, artist, engineer and visionary teacher; died 30 April 1993.

'I want my funeral to be truly ecumenical, bringing together my Orthodox roots with the love and inspiration I have found in CARA* and with my partner David (Rev. David Randall). Through my journey with HIV from the dark to the light, I have known the spiritual power of love to combat fear.'

CARA, Care and Resources for People Affected by HIV/AIDS, was launched in 1988 by David Randall, an Anglican priest, as a response in pastoral ministry towards those affected in whatever way by HIV/AIDS.

Father Gordon Twist talking with Leon at his home after giving him communion. Leon is HIV-positive. Father Gordon is a Roman Catholic priest working full-time for CARA, an ecumenical pastoral ministry for people affected by AIDS and HIV which has been operating in West London since 1988.

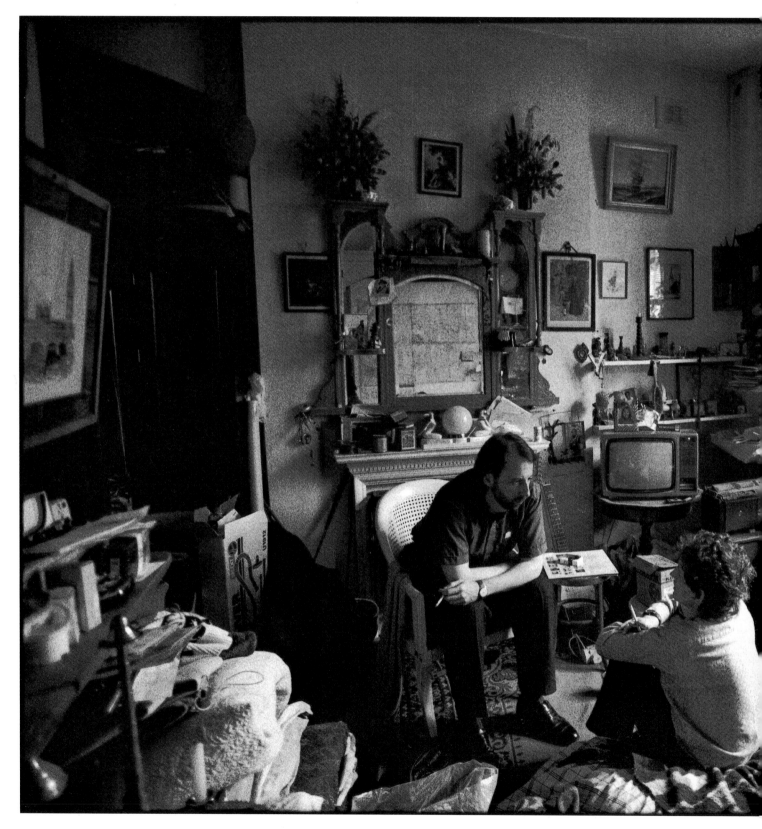

Father Jonathan French talking to friends of Danny Barrett after holding a memorial service for Danny at the London Lighthouse, one year after his death. Danny, though hard of hearing, was a co-founder of Bloolips, a successful drag, singing and dancing show that went on tour around the world.

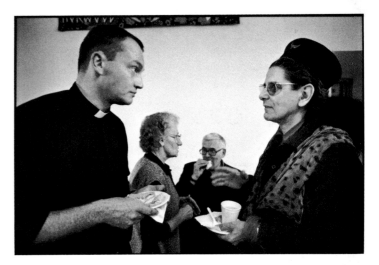

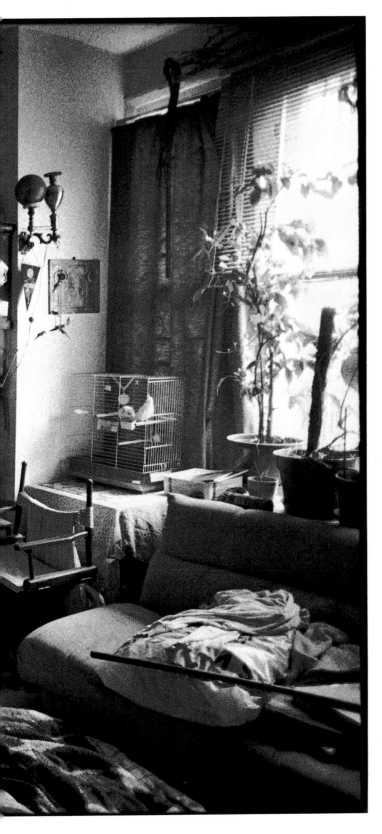

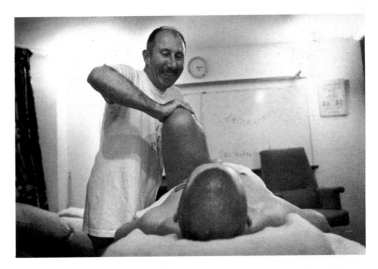

Terry King providing massage at CARA for Steve Kuliczkowski who was diagnosed as HIV-positive eight years ago. Terry describes his massage as holistic or self-healing as it provides relief from stress and increases circulation. Terry feels that this increase in circulation promotes the growth of red blood cells, makes clients aware that their body can fight the virus and puts them in a frame of mind to want to do it. Steve says, 'I have been coming here for massage since October 1992. I had complete liver failure and the hospital said I only had days to live. But in my own mind, no way was I going to die – I had too many loose ends. After an operation I went to the London Lighthouse. I was very weak. There was a cancellation for massage. Massage took away the tension and stress, which helped a lot. I am much stronger now. It helps put my problems into perspective.'

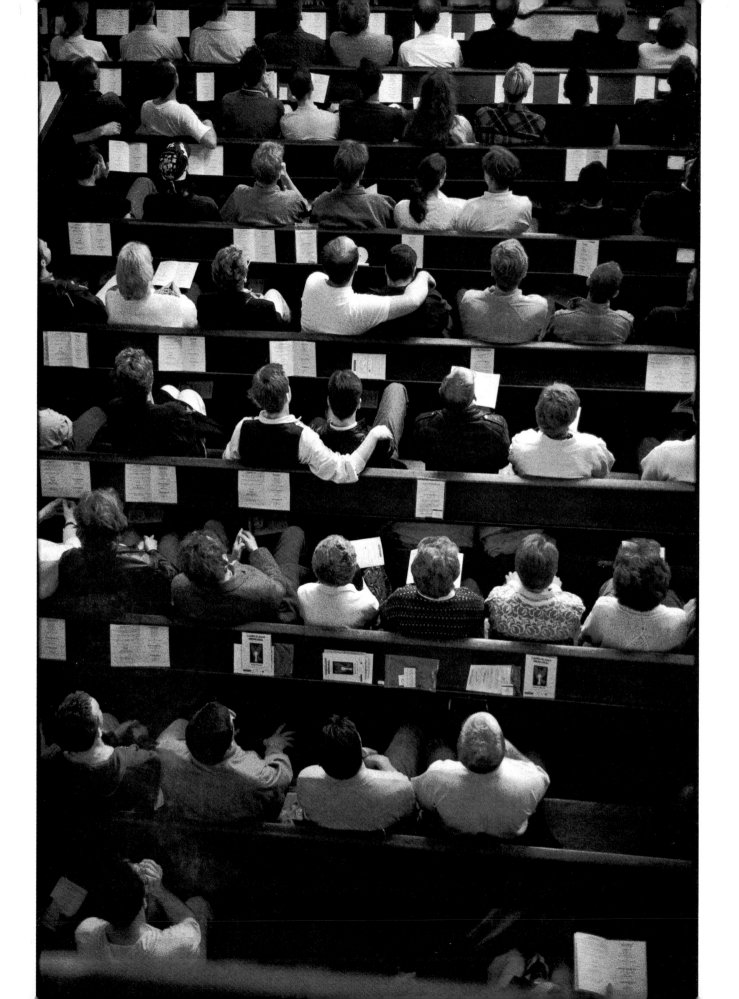

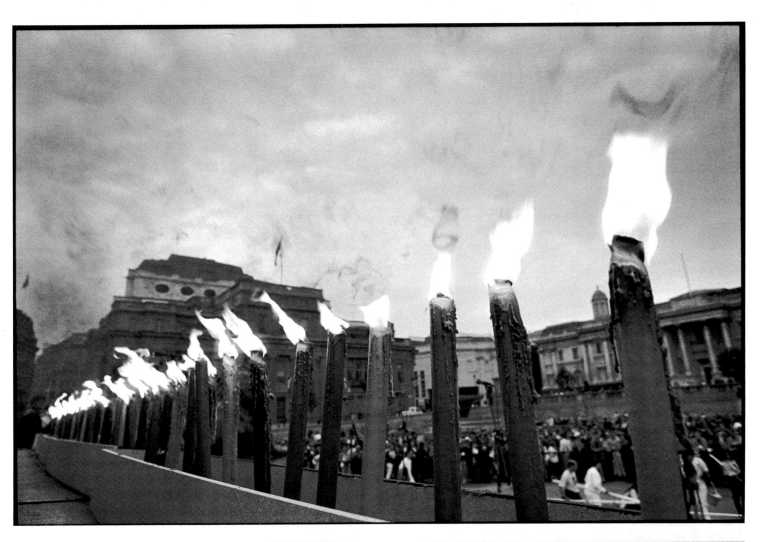

Candles burn at Trafalgar Square for the 1993 Candlelight Memorial, held to demonstrate international solidarity with people living with HIV and AIDS. Similar memorials were held in over 250 cities around the world.

People attending the Remembrance Service at St Martin-in-the-Fields after the 1993 Candlelight Memorial.

Viewing Memorial Quilts at St Martin-in-the-Fields at the end of the 1993 Remembrance Service.

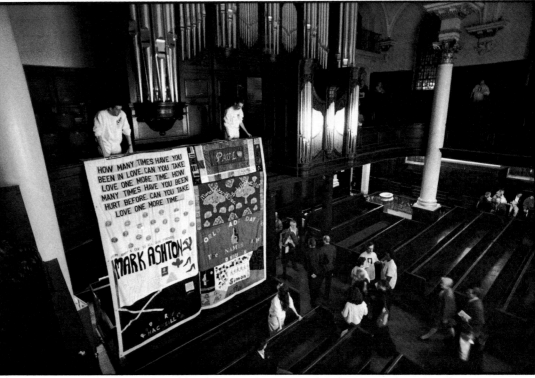

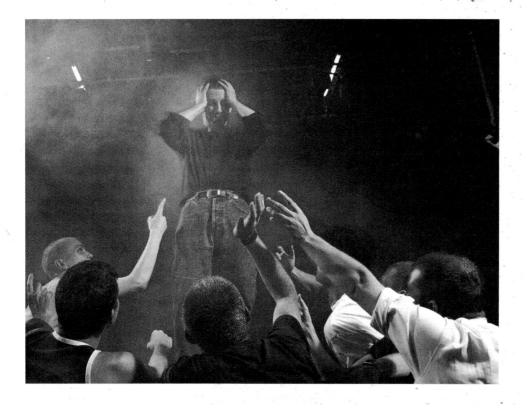

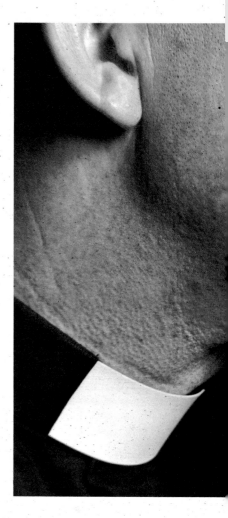

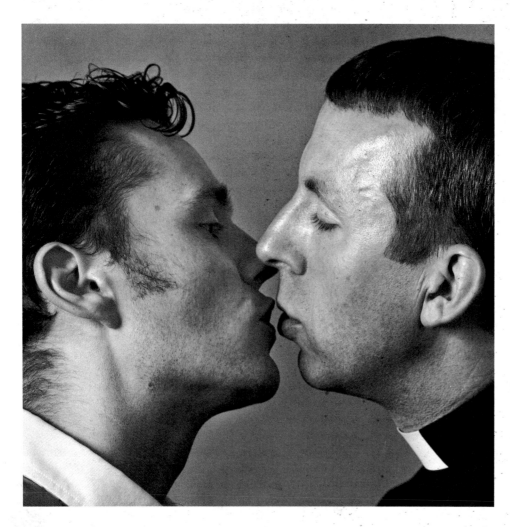

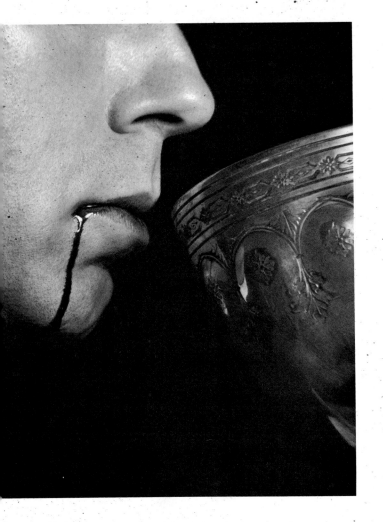
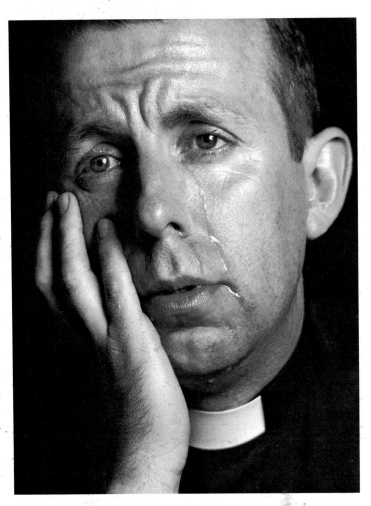

MARTIN HAZELL

'The AIDS crisis came to me first when I was called to a house where a family was grieving for a son who had died with AIDS. It was 1985 and the family had the multiple grief of being ostracized by their church and unable to find an undertaker. We met, that family and I, and my journey began . . .

'When I became a National AIDS Advisor to the United Reformed Church in 1987, the church's concern centred on the fear of contamination through sharing the communion cup. The church wanted to learn – like everyone else they were afraid; they sought me out to teach and be with them. I was loved and supported by many in the church. But some hid their fear behind anger. I received hate mail and a series of threatening phone calls – life-threatening phone calls. A holy kiss, a sign of love, became a Judas kiss, an encounter with fear.

'Once I was asked to lead prayers in a gay night-club – appropriately named "Heaven". Imagine a clergyman there when all around wanted to dance! I was embarrassed and the words stuck in my throat. A few hecklers made me wish the dance floor would swallow me up.

'I have known literally hundreds of people with AIDS – not saints, not sinners either, but people. I have loved them. I have watched their spirits soar; I have watched them fall apart. I have been there at their successes; I have been there when they got sick. I have held them when they died.

'At funerals, there are so many naked emotions. The family is bereft, not understanding why their son never came home. Confused: who are these other people? Friends. Friends who had become family. Friends kissing, loving and supporting each other – isn't that family? Is this what it means to be gay? Sometimes families understand, sometimes not. Friends look at the family and understand why their friend never went home. They look at the family and see strangers. And I am in the middle. Holding the balance and making sure that one group does not take over.

'This journey is indeed long and arduous. On my way, I have found love from those whom society rejects. I have found a new church; intimate with raw emotion – a richness like tasting the blood of Christ.'

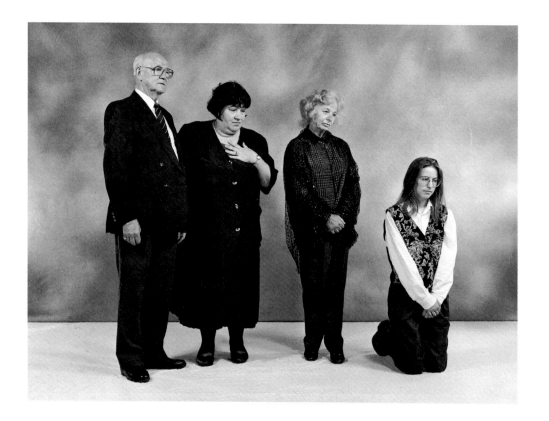
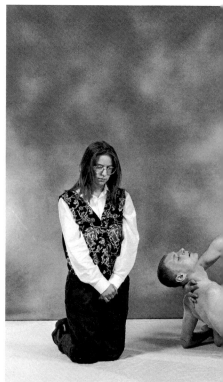

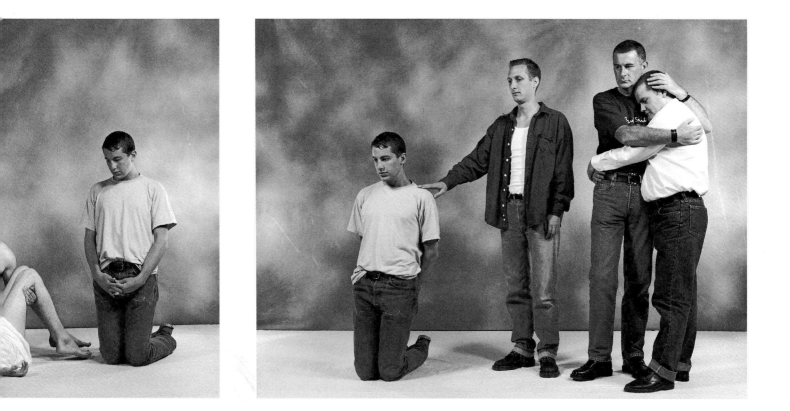

CHAPTER 5

BUDDIES

Photographs by Judah Passow

A Buddy is a specially trained volunteer who is paired with a person with AIDS. Buddies help with everyday tasks like shopping, but most importantly, they offer emotional support in a way that social services, and often family and friends, cannot.

Stories of Buddies frequently involve personal crisis, but they are stories of strength too; strength of the person with AIDS, the strength of the Buddy and the strength of the relationship. The intimate bond that develops between the two reveals aspects of personal growth as well as the despair that often accompanies all the difficulties and loss.

FRANK AND LOUISE

Extract from Louise's diary:

Saturday 24 November 1990.
Met Frank for the first time. Delightful fellow. Gave me tea, cakes and wine. Invited him out for dinner at local restaurant off Abbey Road.

'All his working life, Frank had been a highly respected costumier at the National Theatre and at Bermans. On one of our last outings he was wearing one of his great suits, a Prince of Wales check. We went to a brasserie for lunch and sat outside. This gentle, light April day was one of the best of many we enjoyed together and made up, to some extent, for the really black and awful moments he suffered.

'Although we talked about absolutely everything, I couldn't ever ask Frank if he was afraid of death and dying. He'd got hold of a copy of *Exit*, so we did discuss suicide. But we knew he really had no intention of killing himself – he said he just liked to know what his options were.

'I asked Frank once if he didn't resent, even hate, having to be so nice to all the "helpers", "carers", nurses, doctors and to me etc. (The boys and girls at Tresham were lovely to him, as was everyone at St Mary's and Mildmay.) He admitted that yes, he sometimes did. But only very, very rarely, considering everything, was Frank ever demanding or rude and who could bloody well blame him? And then he'd *always* phone to say, "Sorry".

'Not that Frank didn't do as much as he could for himself. He even learned to administer his medication via a Hickman Line and, later, by Portacath – both fiendishly difficult procedures; so daily he prevented himself from going blind.'

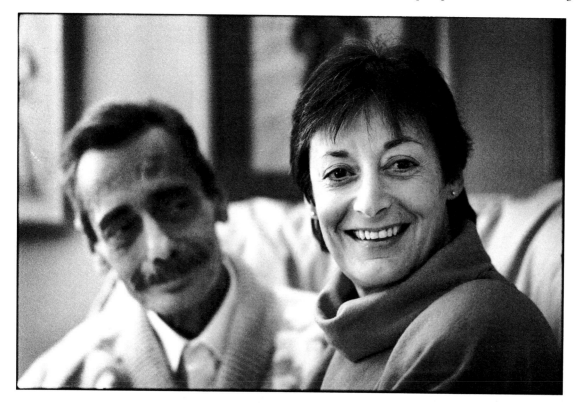

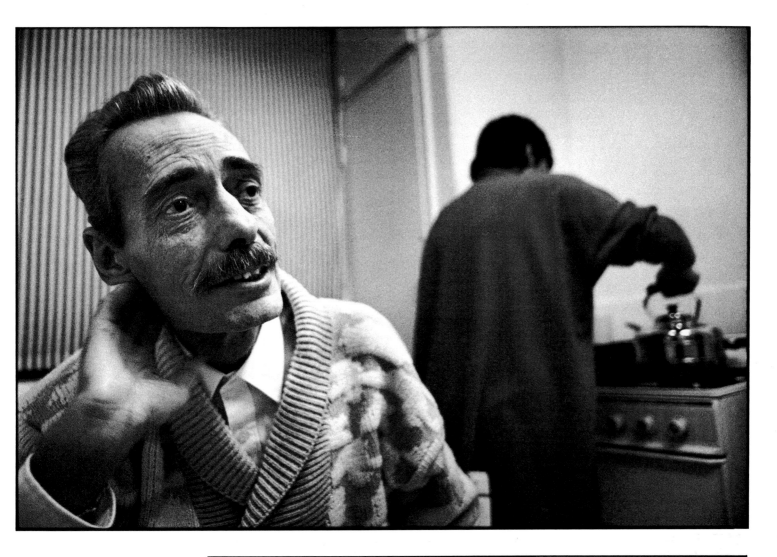

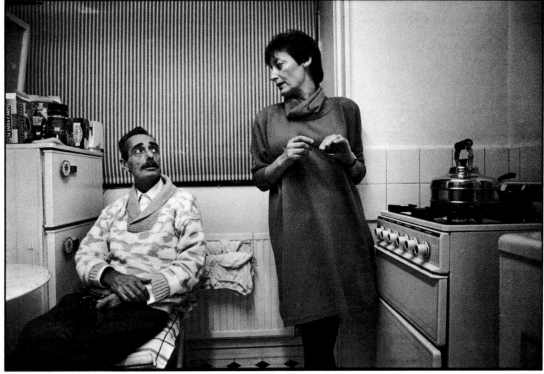

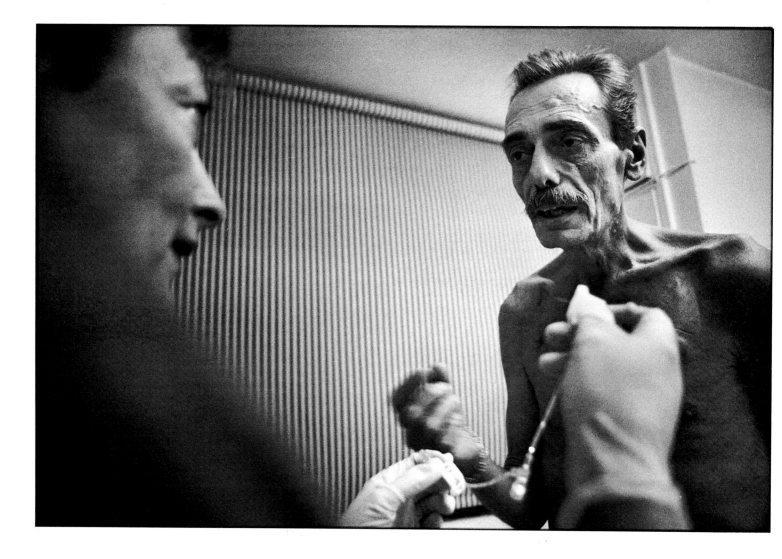

Extract from Louise's diary:

Wednesday 10 June 1991.
Frank died fifteen minutes after midnight – Thursday, I suppose;
and I'm glad I was with him.

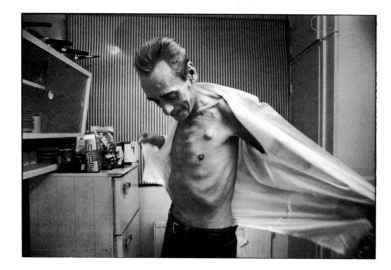

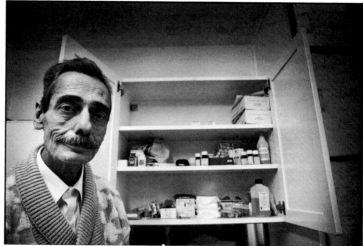

F AND KATHERINE

Katherine supported F through the many ups and downs of her engagement and wedding. The path of this true love had not been easy, with anxious speculation about the outcome right up to the point when rings were exchanged.

'Six years ago I was diagnosed as HIV-positive, then I became aware that I had a little guest in my blood, a tiny element which would try to eat my defences away and so threaten my life. I declared war, then I decided I would be the winner and after six years, I am still well. I have never been in hospital as an inpatient, and I have coped with many of the nasty emotional and psychological repercussions of being diagnosed as HIV-positive.

'I got married about a month ago. I did it out of love and so did the man who decided to marry me. We are thinking now of children; it is risky but we are not ruling it out of discussion straightaway. I am sure that if our faith in life is strong enough we could have a healthy child – we probably will do.'

F, May 1993

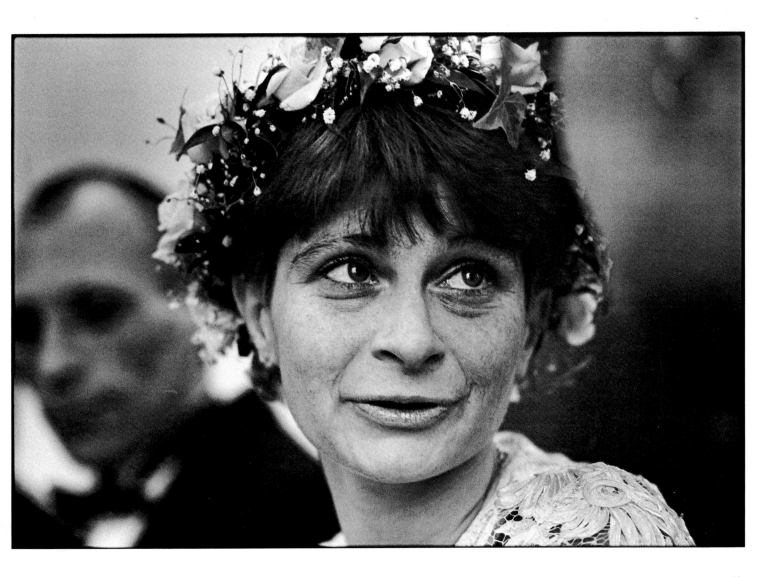

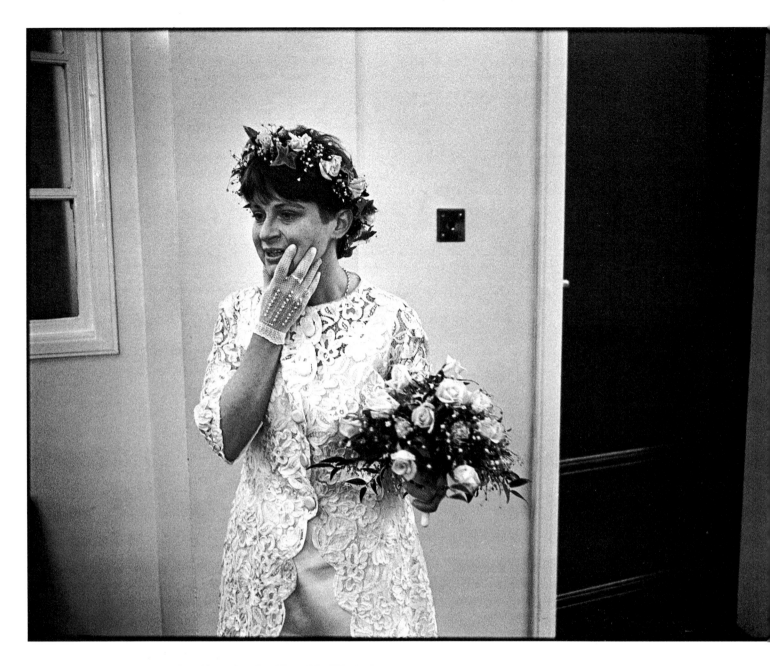

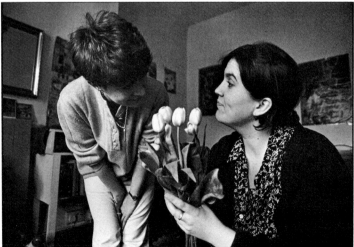

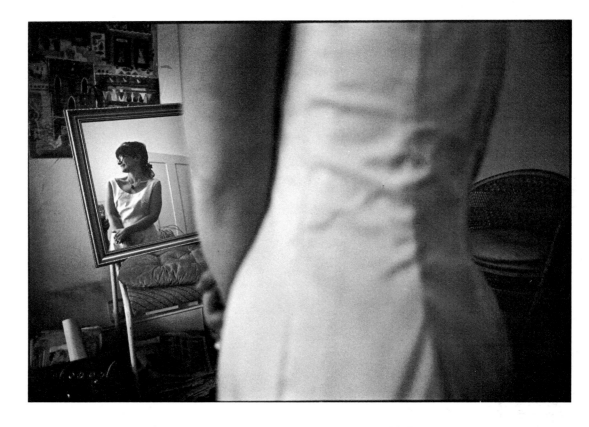

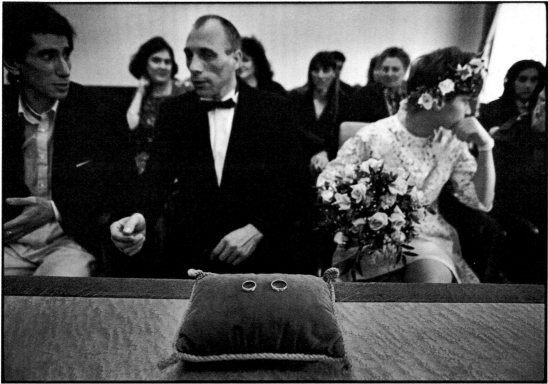

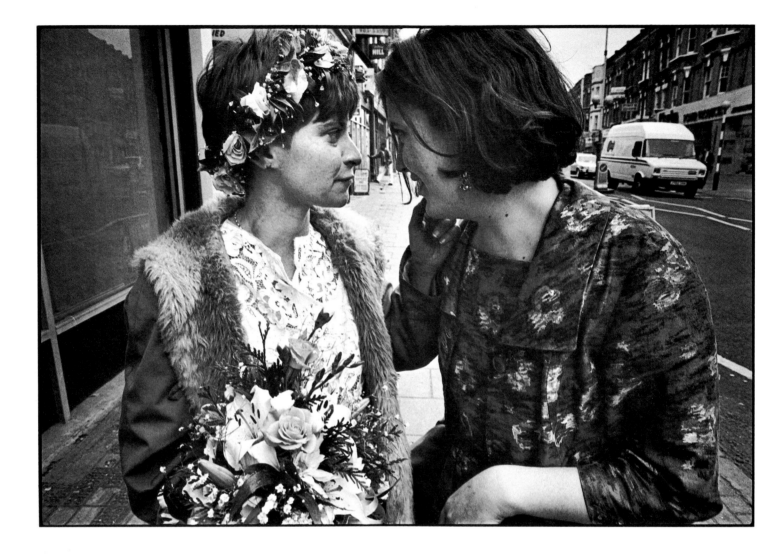

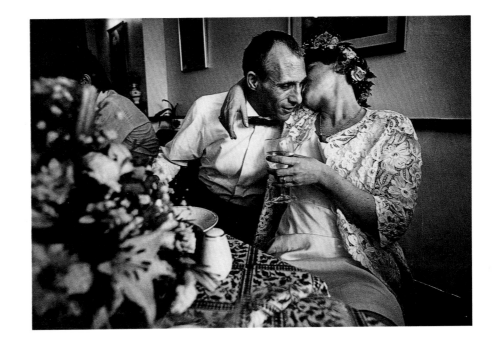

CHAPTER 6

GRIEF AND LOSS

Photographs by Mark Power

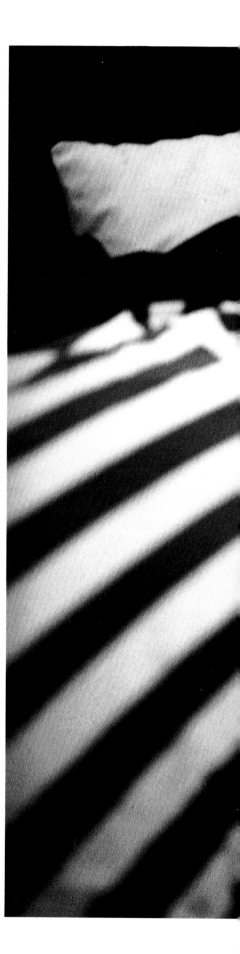

Most of us assume that someone, somewhere, will grieve for our death. We hope that those who knew us will be able to cope with the pain of loss. The death of a loved one with AIDS can leave particular scars. Discovering the cause of death sometimes means losing more than a physical presence, shattering long-held illusions which elicit a distressing mixture of love and anger. Lack of comprehension about the illness, allied to the shock that it could intrude so brutally into ordinary life, causes unique suffering. In a largely unknowing, yet judgemental, society this cause of death can be discreetly ignored or, at worst, denied.

TIM AND RICARDO

'They had a memorial at the hospital for him the week before last. They wanted to do something for him. We basically said, "Whatever you want to do is appropriate", because it wasn't really for him, it was for them. But we did say it wouldn't be appropriate for them to do something religious, because he was totally unreligious – he didn't have any kind of belief in that way at all. So they had it . . . and of course it *was* a religious thing, which I thought was a bit of a sham.

'But the really good thing about it was that a lot of people made tributes to him. They said some incredibly nice things about him, although it hurt a little that they didn't mention how he died, or that he was gay. It was upsetting to have to think about it so intensely for that length of time.

'The cremation was at Golders Green and was a non-religious event. Basically, we just played some music, then I got up and said something over some other music, then Helen gave a reading followed by some more music, and that was it.

'It was very difficult because, apart from saying that he wanted to be cremated, his other wishes weren't written down.

'We'd discussed it, of course, but all he'd said was "As far as I'm concerned, once I've gone I've gone, and you might as well chuck me in the river", which of course we couldn't do. There seemed to be a lot of pressure for a funeral, but he wouldn't have wanted that at all. He didn't want any fuss and people said that, in the end, we got it just about right.

'I took three roses, a red, a pink and a yellow. The reason I took the three is actually really stupid . . . it's a bit embarrassing . . . but it was one from me and one from each of the cats. Afterwards I took the roses to the little park where his mother's tree is, and I put them there. I think they've now finally gone. But they were there for quite a long time.

'I often wonder about some of the little things that he said and did in those few days before he went into hospital for the last time – whether he knew what was happening. As he walked out of the

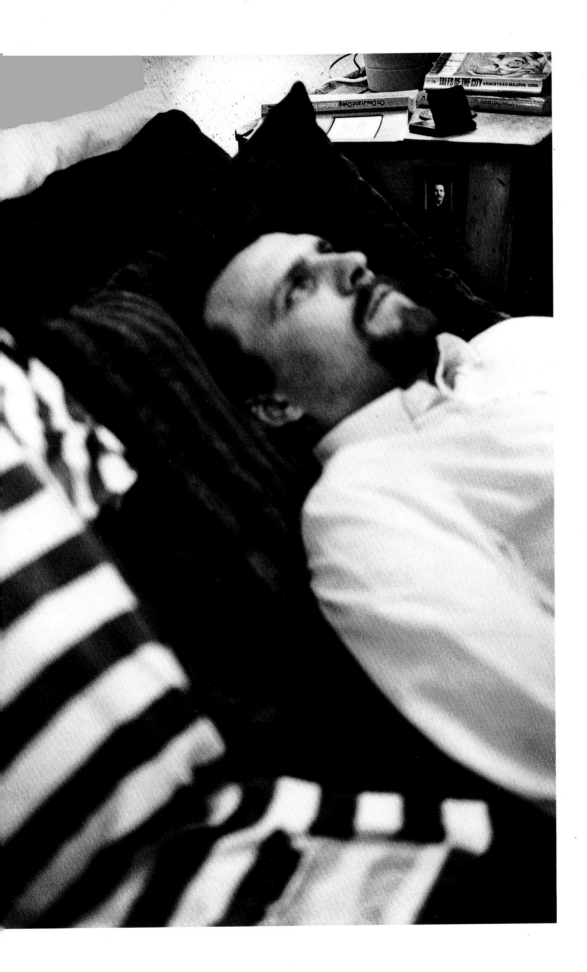

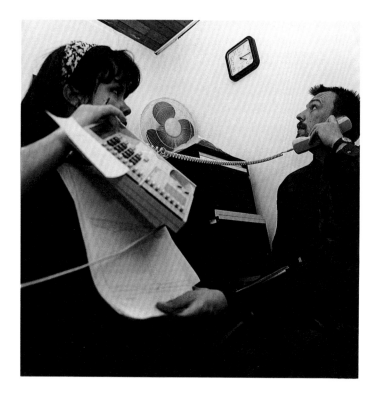

flat and we went out of the front door, he said "Don't let the flat go to pot".

'We first met at the London Apprentice pub on Old Street in 1988. I came home here with him. I don't really know what happened, but basically I never left. We met on the 22nd of August, and I officially moved in in November, but in that time there was only one night when I didn't stay here.

'So in effect, I moved in straightaway. I sort of knew that it was going to happen. It wasn't anything corny like love at first sight, but I just think that sometimes you know these things when you feel very comfortable with someone.

'About six weeks after we met, we planned a holiday in Madrid. Around that time, the subject just came up. I said, "Have you had a test?", and he said "Yes", so I said "What was it?", and he said "Oh, it was positive", and then he laughed. At first I thought he was joking. We talked about it a bit, but at the time it was something I was still quite naïve about. I didn't yet know anyone who was positive and there are still a lot of people who don't – in this country the worst is still to come.

'I don't think I thought he was going to die. It wasn't until the day before he died . . . I think that's when I finally acknowledged to myself that it was going to happen.

'Whenever he got ill in any way I would always encourage him to go to the hospital or do something about it, but he resisted. I don't mean he resisted treatment, but he'd often delay getting things done. He'd always rather wait and see if it turned out bad.

'There were periods last year when he'd lie on the sofa week after week with fevers and he'd have to change his nightclothes three times a night because he'd be soaked in sweat. He'd shake and shake and shake for periods of about forty minutes, then he'd get hot and then incredibly cold. It was very difficult to live with that, not doing anything about it, but it always had to be his decision, and he'd always just wait and see. It took a lot before he would do anything, and it was the same the last time. Still, I don't think it would have done a great deal of good anyway, knowing what eventually happened.

'It's a very selfish thing to say, but I'd rather have him here ill than not at all, even though he loathed being ill, and he had one or two bouts of real depression. Now I haven't got those things, I've either got to find other things to distract me or I've got to face up to what's happened – and that's a difficult thing to do.

'Initially there's shock or disbelief. When someone dies there are an incredible number of things to do. So much comes through the letterbox demanding attention and that's a distraction. Then, after all that was over, I think I over-compensated and I went out an awful lot. Fridays and Saturdays I'd stay out until the early hours, because I hated being here. I'd do anything not to be here. I certainly didn't like having people round, but I didn't really want to go out with other people either – there's an awkwardness – they don't know what to do or say.

'I've changed nothing about the flat. Even stupid things . . . on the bed we had three pillows each, and his were much better than mine. I've got the three flattest pillows, but I can't bring myself to replace them with the ones on his side. Things like that I just don't do, but I've obviously got to get over it at some point. I don't know if I'm doing it just so I don't have to face up to it . . . I still

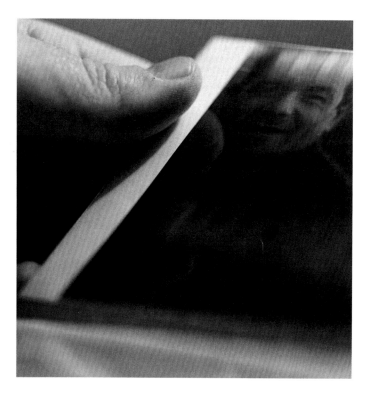

keep his T-shirt on the bed, over his pillow. It was my favourite T-shirt of his. So many of the photos I've got are of him wearing that shirt. It's something that I associate with him completely. When he went into hospital for the last time he had a lot of blood transfused as he was incredibly anaemic. They gave him pints and pints of blood. One day they were changing the drip and they spilt some over that shirt. They took it off and said they'd get the laundry people to clean it. I think that was on the Wednesday and he died on the Friday. Events overtook me, and I forgot about the shirt. But after he died they asked me if I wanted to pick out something for him to wear, and I was really torn over that shirt. I wanted to keep it for myself, even though I really associated it with him, but it wasn't there. The next day I went back and they'd got all his stuff together, and the T-shirt was back from the laundry. Anyway, now it's there on the side of the bed where he slept but it can't stay there forever though. I know I'll have to do something with it eventually.

'There are times when, for no reason at all, I can feel very upset. Very stupid and bizarre things trigger it off, like, for example, Cilla Black's *Surprise! Surprise!* show. Watching things like that, even though I know they're so contrived, it's really difficult not to get emotional. I know it's a load of old rubbish, but it just sets me off. I actually find weekends very difficult.

'People have a fear of bringing up the subject – I think they think it'll be upsetting for you. People say "You look after yourself . . ." and it's very loaded with meaning. They can't seem to bring themselves to say anything else, and that's really difficult, because that's really all I think about all the time, but I'm also very aware that it's not what everyone else thinks about.

'I'm only 27, I could have another 50 years ahead of me, and yet the person who I wanted to share that time with isn't going to be here. That's something I find very difficult to understand.

'Our relationship went to another level when he became ill. You're forced to have a much greater understanding of someone. I was 22 when I met him, and he shaped the person I am today. He was the motivation for everything I did.

'Undoubtedly he was positive because he was around during a very liberating time for gay men, the 1970s, the first time when there was any kind of openness about it. Homosexuality was only legalized at the end of the 1960s. But to say that seems to imply that he almost deserved it, but no one deserves it, no one does, it's a horrible thing to watch someone die in that way.

'I don't care who they are or what they've done – no one deserves it.'

Tim

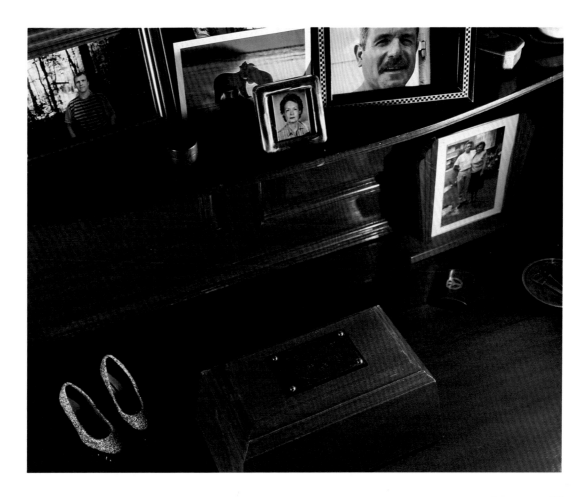

REG AND DOREEN LANGBRIDGE

'It's two years on 12 April. It's getting harder if anything. We still look at his photograph sometimes and think it's impossible, it can't have happened. To think that we'll never see him again. He was such a live-wire, always making us laugh. We've laughed with him, cried with him, suffered with him. He was all of our life.'

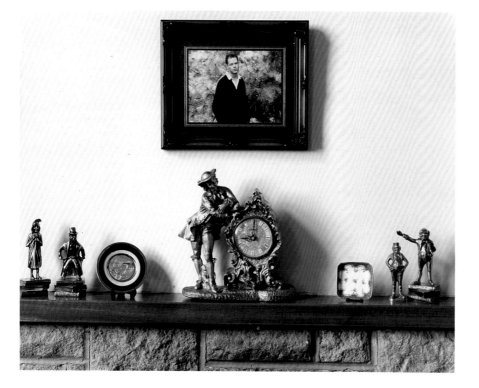

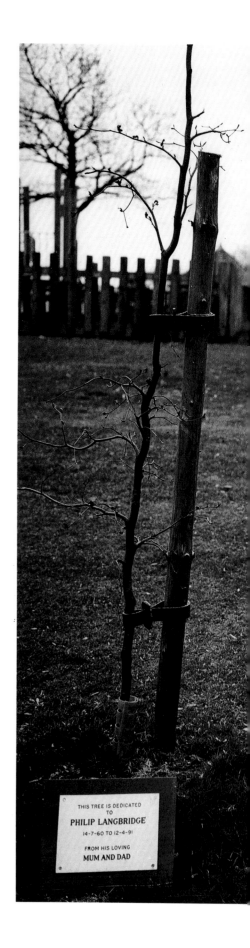

THIS TREE IS DEDICATED
TO
PHILIP LANGBRIDGE
14-7-60 TO 12-4-91

FROM HIS LOVING
MUM AND DAD

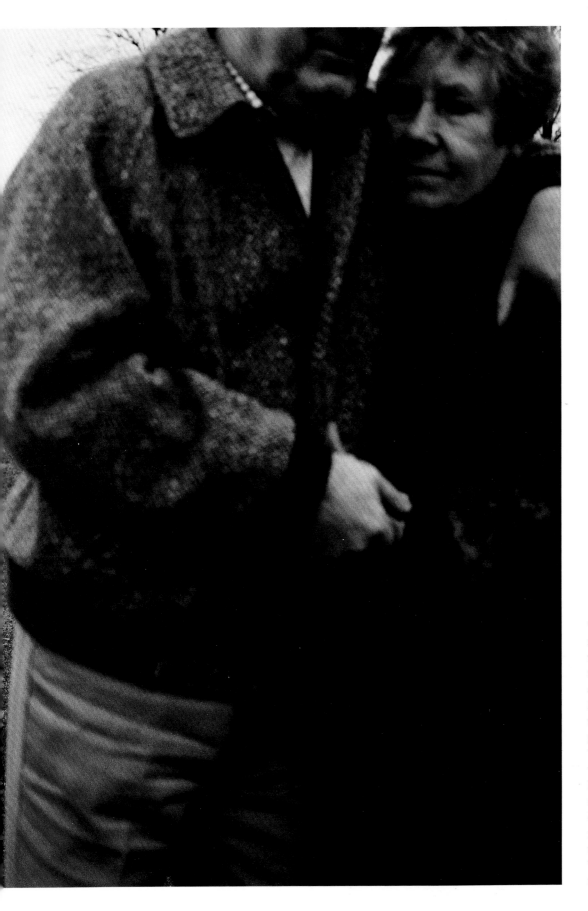

'Whenever those silly scare-
mongering pamphlets came
through the door, we just used
to tear them up and throw them
away. It just wasn't going to
happen to our family, even
though we knew our son was
gay, it never entered our minds.
We know now what people mean
when they say they have a broken
heart. We know what it's like
ourselves. I feel it's true that you
can die of a broken heart, because
you get so low that you just want
to die. Part of your life has gone.
You're not complete anymore. We
feel it so badly.'

'We had a bit of a thing about shells. About half of them were picked by Philip when he went to Indonesia for the first time. That's when he fell in love with the place. Then there are others that we got in Indonesia when we went there together. Others I used to buy Philip when he went into hospital for his blood transfusions and tests. While he was coming round from his anaesthetic, I used to pop out and buy him a little pressie for being a good lad, so I'd often buy him a shell. I bought the "forget-me-not" after Philip died . . . it seemed fab that it said what it did.

'Philip always said that he wanted his ashes sprinkled in Chiswick Park. On the first anniversary of his death I really felt that I should do something with them. I got up really early and went out there. It was a beautiful sunny day and not at all sad. I was expecting it to be, but it was lovely.

'I scattered half the ashes on the water from the bridge, and the other half I planted in the ground. It was something that I wanted to do on my own. Philip actually wanted me to do it on my own as he didn't really want a ceremony or anything.

'He was sitting up, but he was somewhere else, and semi-conscious I suppose. I asked the others if they minded going out for a while, because I needed to be on my own with Philip. So I was talking to Philip – I never knew if it was the drugs or the illness – but he could hardly talk, and his mouth didn't move when he was talking. I don't remember exactly what I was talking about, but I do remember saying to him that if he was ready to die that it was all right by me, and that I obviously didn't want him to die, but if he was ready, then it was fine. I was holding his hand and he was sort of clenching it. Then I told him that I loved him

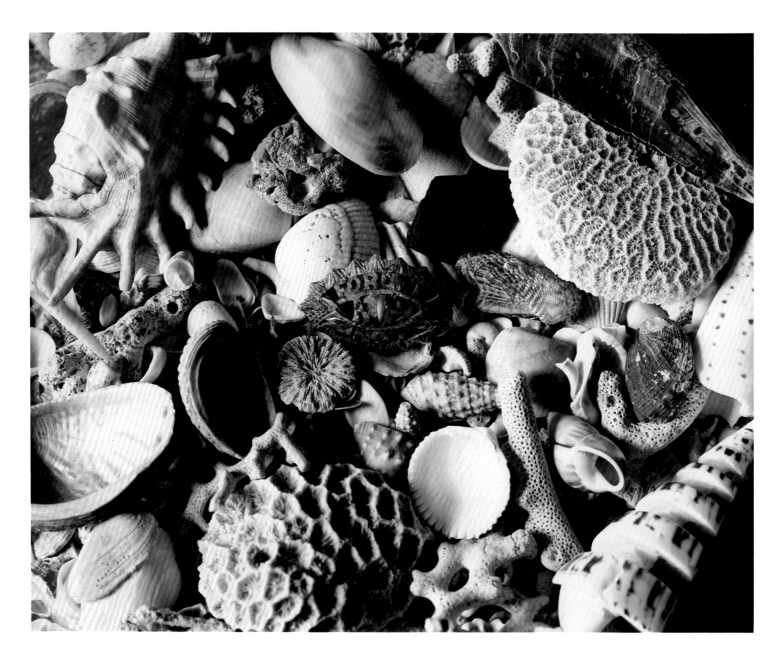

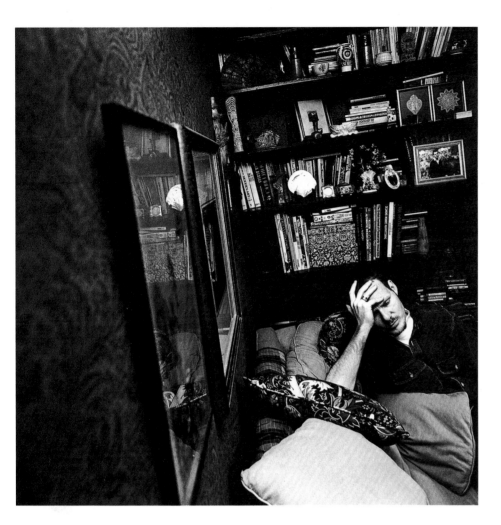

and I remember that he had that little smile on his face and he said back really quietly, "I love you too," and then he sort of coughed and just stopped.

'There was a tiny, tiny part of me that realized that he'd died, but most of me couldn't think that. The nurse came in, took his pulse, and she said, "He's gone". I remember I gave out this horrendous sort of yelp, a scream. I can hear myself doing it now.

'A lot's happened in the two years since Philip died. I was just sort of left. I hadn't got a job and I hadn't got Philip to look after. It was sort of unreal having time on my hands with nothing to do. For probably two years before he died we spent twenty-four hours a day together, every day. He *was* my best friend. We had close friends, but even so we relied on each other. My whole life had been Philip. My job, my career, had just been shoved out of the way – out of choice – and *my* life was *our* life together. Then all of a sudden he wasn't here anymore, so I didn't really have a life anymore.

'People did rally round and were wonderful, but whatever anybody could have done for me could never have been enough. I didn't want them really, I wanted Philip, but he wasn't here anymore.

'After Philip died, I started getting quite sick and lots of physical things kept going wrong. I was relentlessly at the doctors.

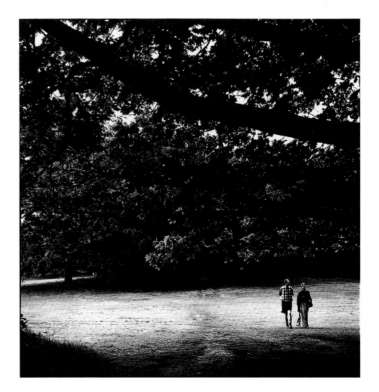

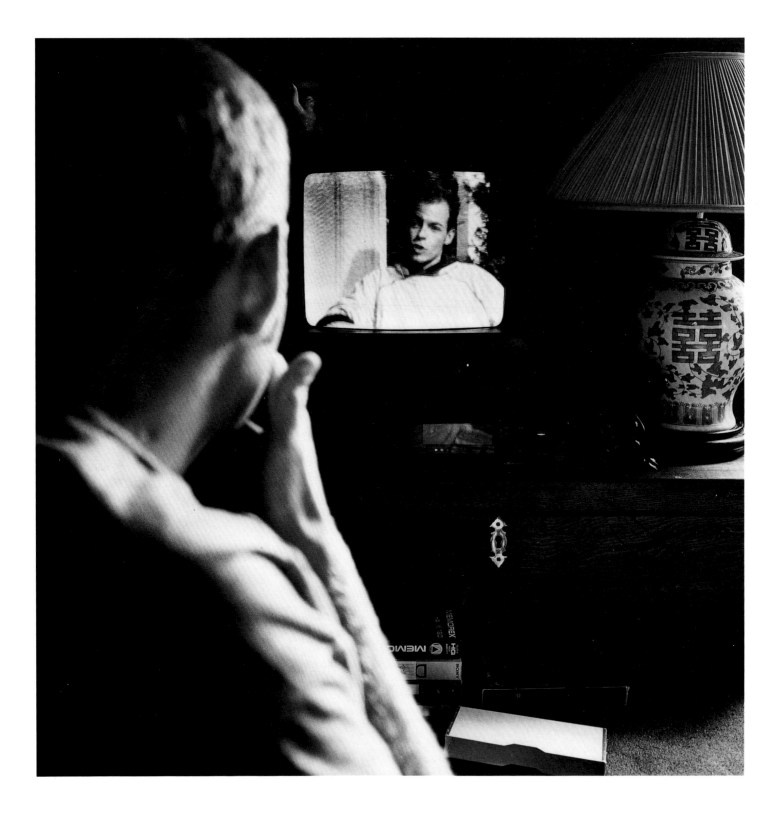

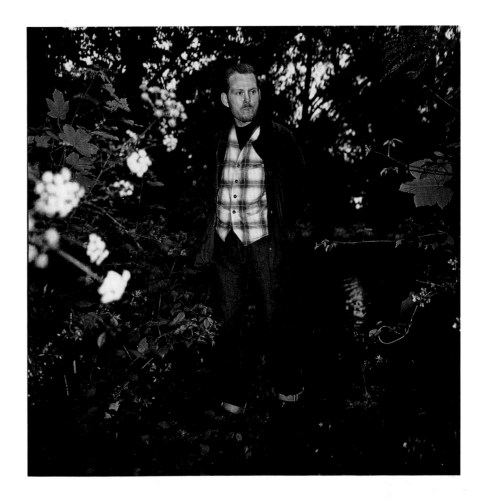

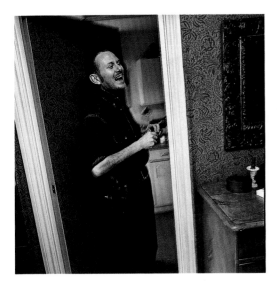

'At one point about four months after Philip died, I thought that I was cracking up. It was stress of course. One day I got up and I was physically shaking. I was petrified, I didn't know what was wrong.

'I was put on anti-depressants for about nine months. The physical problems went away. Since then it's been up and down all the time. At Christmas I was put back on them, and I finished taking them last week. I feel OK at the moment.

'Things do change though. I've had some good times in the last two years too. Times when I've felt really good and happy. Certainly life goes on – I have a job now, which is very demanding and takes up a lot of my time, and I've met some new people who are nice, and I like the people I work with.

'This was our flat – we moved into it together. We got it together between ourselves. It still feels like it's ours, but Philip is not here anymore, so it doesn't feel helpful to be here. Everything in the flat has a memory, and I love it for that, but it also breaks my heart sometimes. I can't do anything to change the flat, so the only thing I can do is move on.

'I'll always have those memories, and I'll always be in love with Philip, and that'll go with me wherever I am. But I need to move somewhere new and start making a life again, because I don't feel I have yet. My job takes up too much of my time, and the rest of the time I don't do much, so it feels my life is not very productive.'

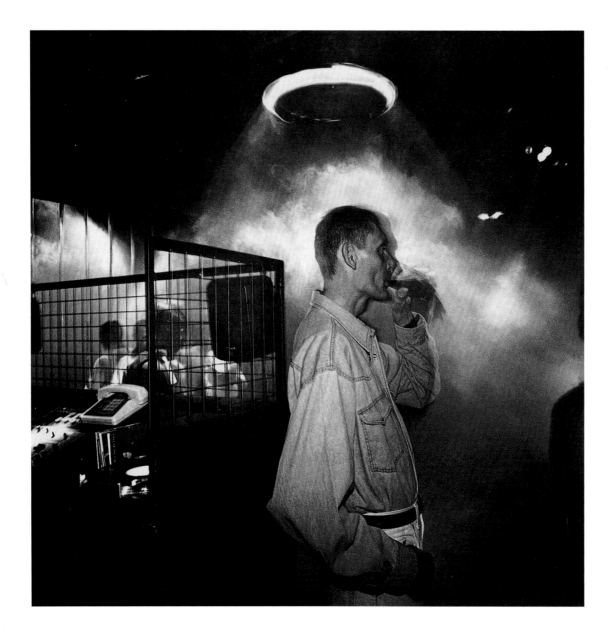

KEN

'When I had pneumonia and I was bored in hospital someone suggested I do some needlework. I thought about it and decided to embroider a cloth with people's names on it. That was about four years ago. Now there are about 120 or 130 names on it, all people who've passed through "Open Door" at some time.

'It must be – with people I know from all over the country, not just from Brighton – 170, yes, it must be about 170.

'I was classed as a professional funeral-goer because I went to nearly all of them, but it's my way of saying goodbye to friends. I did get to the stage where I thought that I couldn't cry anymore, but then you find that some are really hard. Maybe the partners felt left out of it. But some have been spiritually uplifting, because nowadays, instead of everyone always wearing black, quite often

everyone wears bright colours. At one of them I went to, we all let go of coloured balloons. You could see the balloons drifting off to heaven.

'Sometimes I get very shaky when I go to funerals, like one last year. I went to someone's funeral whose name was Ken, and it kept going through my mind that it was like my own funeral. It was a strange experience.

'Sometimes I'm at a funeral and I think back to other people who I've known . . . perhaps I hadn't been able to let go at their funeral so I do later at someone else's.

'Most of them have been younger than me, and often I feel guilty: why am I still going when they have gone? I've been told not to think that but I still do.

'There were three in one day once. And there's been other days when there's been more than one. Going back, about five years ago when I was doing hospital visits, five died in one week. It seems to go in cycles. That does get you down a little bit.

'I was diagnosed by a doctor who did a test without telling me. It was about eight or nine years back, I've lost touch with exactly when. I know it was June but that's all I can remember.

'I had to decide whether or not to tell my mum and dad. I felt that in the end that it would be more of a shock if anything were to happen to me and they found out that way. So I did tell them. At least they'd be prepared to cope with it nearer the time. My mum had guessed that something was wrong. She said, "You've got it, haven't you?" and the next thing I heard was the phone banging against the wall, and her screaming down the phone "He's got it! He's got it!" Ever since then, I've had a lot of support from my family.

'We were told not to talk about it because of the way the press were handling it then, but I decided to be open about it and tell everyone right from the start. I wasn't rejected by anyone, so I was lucky. But when I was at a rehabilitation centre recovering from my brain operation, I had to have my own knife and fork, my own basin and everything. I remember cutting my finger one day while I was peeling the spuds, and they threw them all away!

'I do get bouts of depression now and again, but instead of letting AIDS and HIV suffocate me, I suffocate it. I don't wake up with it on my mind anymore like I used to. When I used to see the word AIDS anywhere, on an advert or something, it used to hit me like a ton of bricks. That doesn't happen anymore. You can guarantee that everyday you hear the word somewhere or other. Yes, sometimes it does still get me down a bit.

'You go through anger . . . depression . . . before you come to accept it and with the arthritis as well I kept thinking that I was jinxed.

'When I was in my teens and I couldn't cope with the pain of the arthritis and finding out that I was gay too, I tried to kill myself. Because I was under age, the hospital had to tell my parents *why* I tried to kill myself.

'I ended up having electric shock treatment for about six months to try and turn me straight. They thought that they could cure it. I had these electrodes attached to me, mainly to my arms, and they'd show me photographs of men, and I had to – mentally – get myself aroused. They gave me a list to follow: meeting him, getting home with him, undressing him, then going to bed, and then just as I got to the erotic part in my mind they gave me an electric shock and showed me pictures of women. They had to put the voltage up each week because it wasn't doing anything.

'In the end I asked my parents if they wanted me to be happy or miserable all my life. I said that pretending to be straight when I knew I wasn't was making me ill. On the last day of the electric shock treatment I was on my way home, standing at the bus stop when I met someone, and I went off with him for the night . . . and that's where it all started!

'The last relationship I had was was ten or eleven years ago, and that was only for about six months. Previous to that it was about another ten years.

'I do get very lonely sometimes and often I wish I had a partner.

'I've told my mum and dad that if ever I do get a partner, and anything should happen to me, don't cut him out, because he'll need support as well. I've seen it happen to so many other people.

'Other times I feel that I don't want a partner, because I wouldn't like to put him through misery if anything should happen to me. This way I won't hurt anyone and I feel I might be selfish wanting one. But then I feel it would be nice to have someone as moral support, to get a cuddle from them when it ends . . . if it ever comes to that part.

'Most people who were diagnosed at the same time as me have gone now. When "Open Door" started, there were about ten of us. I think that there's only one of them left now. It does make you think that the list is getting shorter and that your name is getting nearer the top.

'A lot of long-term people feel that they don't get the support that they used to get. I was told that I have to think about the new people, about how it was for me when I was first diagnosed, and what they're going through. But long-terms need just as much support, because they're always wondering "How long have we got?"

'We used to really support each other in the old days. The new ones seem to demand a lot more. But sometimes I feel that if it wasn't for us, they wouldn't be getting the benefits now. There was no support for any of us then. When I was diagnosed all those years ago, a group of us just used to meet in someone's front room. I've met a lot of people that I wouldn't have met otherwise if life had been . . . normal.

'Over the years I've been beaten up four times, I think. Ten years after the first attack, after all the blackouts and so on, I finally convinced them that something was wrong, and they gave me the brain operation. Last night I was followed home by a group of men who were singing to the tune of Rod Stewart's *Sailing*, "You are dying, you are dying, you are dying, but we don't care".

'I think I'll write to the Argus about it.'

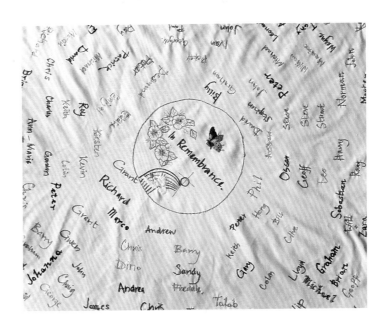

CHAPTER 7

MOTHERS AND CHILDREN

Photographs by Jenny Matthews

Living with HIV, in the intimate relationship that a child shares with its mother or carer, creates extremely intense emotional pressures. None of the contradictory emotions can be rationalized, and both adult and child live on a roller-coaster of love and judgement, support and fear, comfort and alienation. All this is fought on a secret battleground; discretion is essential if the child is to retain contact with the outside world which is not ready to understand what this illness means.

These pictures were inspired by conversations with positive children and positive women and children.

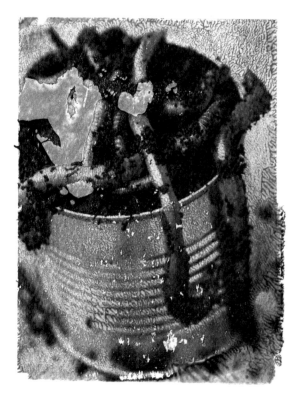

POSITIVE MOTHER

'When my child was a couple of years old her father left me. I was devastated. I felt unloved and unwanted. On holiday I slept with a bisexual gay man. I am now HIV-positive. I feel absolutely no bitterness towards him; it was what I needed at the time.

'I haven't been able to tell my daughter that I'm positive yet. She knows a lot about AIDS from my work with the Trust. She's worn a red ribbon to school, and when her school friends have said that you get AIDS from kissing, she's taken them up on it, but telling her would be giving her a lot to cope with. It's a problem that once people tell one person, even their best friend in confidence, that information is out of your control. Not telling her is difficult too because it implies a lack of trust. I have to think of her emotions though, she associates AIDS with death and has got very angry when friends have died. One of the problems of having a child is coping with the tiredness – having the energy for her as well as for myself, persuading her to help clear up without blackmailing her into doing it because I'm ill.

'We live under a veil of secrecey, getting by with a series of white lies. People often don't want to know, they don't try to put two and two together. When people ask what I do, and I mention the Trust, they assume I'm a doctor or a scientist, they don't want to read between the lines. Sometimes I just want to shout it out, "I'm positive", and other times I just want to withdraw. In the film *Savage Nights,* there's a scene where the woman, knowing that the man is HIV-positive, throws the condom across the room. That sacrificial gesture is so typical of women, "I don't care, I love you." Men are not like that.

'It's very different being a heterosexual woman. You really feel in a minority. For gay men it is no big deal socially to be positive, but because the heterosexual community has not been seriously affected yet, it's much harder for us. If you go out with a new person, there's the question of when you tell them, and how they will react. The normal assumption that people live with is that you have a future, but it's difficult for someone to take on a person who doesn't. You want to live positively, but you also have a life-threatening illness, death comes into it and that changes your relationships. Those who love you often try to deny what's happening – that you'll be different, you'll be all right. It's difficult with children too – normally you assume you'll see them through to adulthood, but I can't do that.'

Caroline

'The media are like a can of worms. We know you want to show what it's like to live with AIDS, but the repercussions for those who are filmed can be devastating. We can't predict what the consequences will be.'

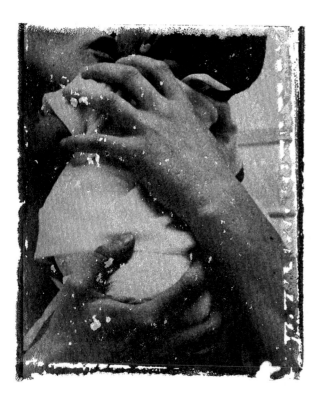

'There are no words to describe
how it feels to tell a whole family
that they are all HIV-positive.'

'I am an HIV counsellor. If I say
what I do at a cocktail party, it's
the kiss of death.'

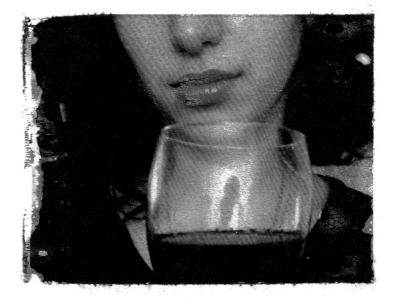

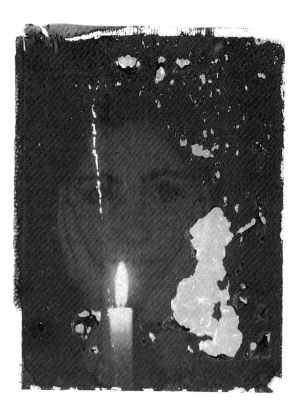

'I know a woman who won't go out. She sits at home with the curtains drawn and the lights out.'

'Telling children passes the burden of secrecy on to them.'

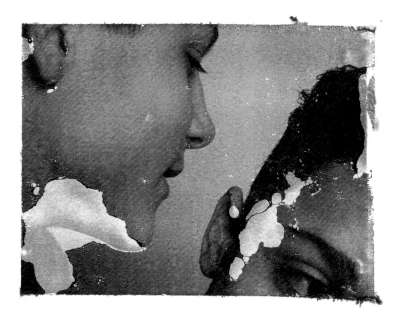

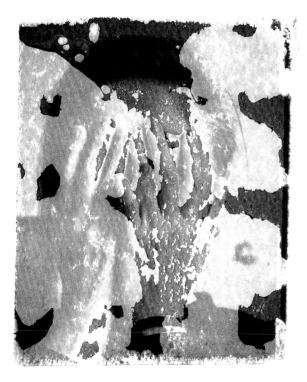

'Overwhelming tiredness. However ill women are, there are still
children to cope with. In practice,
there's no priority for children
because women often can't be
open and say why they need a
place.'

'Any other medical condition you
could talk about. People would be
sympathetic. We live behind a veil
of secrecy.'

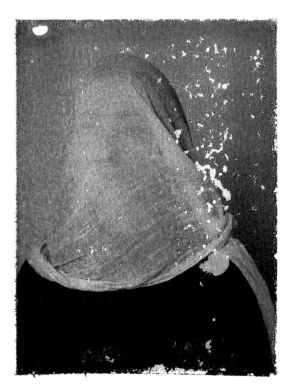

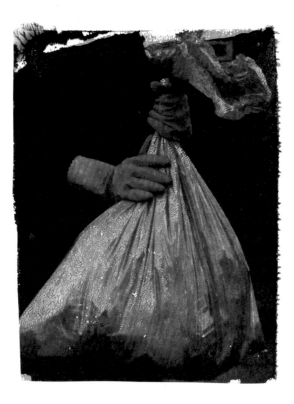

'Mummy, why did the doctor
wear rubber gloves, am I dirty?'

An eleven-year-old draws HIV as a
spider weaving in her lungs.

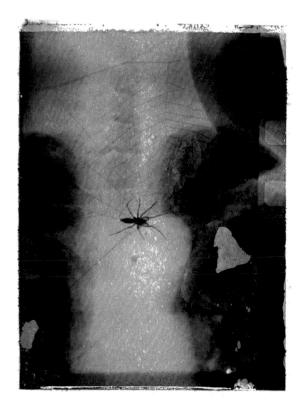

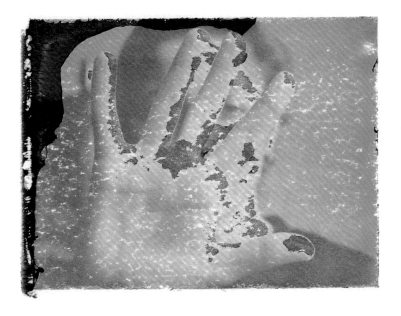

'People are closing down – we're living in a climate of fear.'

'We are talking about real people.'

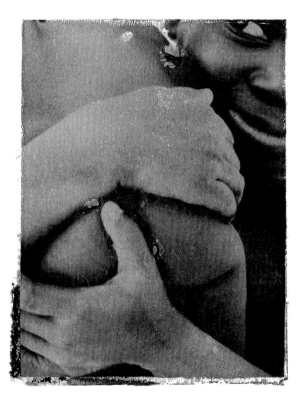

'Three years ago I found out that I was pregnant. A few weeks later my partner told me that he was HIV-positive. For a split second I experienced total fear. I didn't want anything to do with him. I wanted to cut myself off, but a second later I decided to stand by him. As I was carrying his baby and sleeping with him I thought that I was HIV-positive too. It was several months before I knew for sure that I wasn't.

'Some friends know about the HIV, other's don't, but somehow news filters through. By telling them, you're transferring the burden. It's unfair asking people to keep quiet – we need to share the information in order to make sense of it. I've always been open and honest, it's the way I am – my inclination is to tell and share, but when my boyfriend told me he swore me to secrecy, I wasn't to tell anyone – his way of coping was denial and drink.

'All the time it was on the tip of my tongue to tell people. I needed to be heard, I had to tell them for my survival, but I also felt so guilty about breaking my word. I loved and adored him and feared his reaction if he knew that I'd told anyone. In fact, my experiences of telling people were very bad.

'I told my flatmate of the time, but she became very paranoid. She got worried about our toothbrushes being next to each other, and she didn't like me walking around in bare feet – she couldn't cope at all and moved out. I was in the middle of doing my MA, I was pregnant, and since by boyfriend was HIV-positive I thought that I was positive too. I was bursting with this secret. The next friend I told said, "Don't worry, I'll be there for you." And then she disappeared, I didn't see her for the rest of the term. Later she told me she'd set her sights on getting a distinction and couldn't let anything stand in the way of that.

'My child is a miracle and a blessing. If things had happened the other way around, if I'd learnt about the HIV first, she would never have been conceived. As it was, I was thinking I should have an abortion, but then when we knew about the HIV, I couldn't, it was like a last chance to have a child with him, the perfect excuse to try to go on with the pregnancy.

'Eventually I plucked up the courage to tell my mum. She stroked my head – it was the first time she'd done that without making things better – I felt so small.

'My dad didn't speak to me all the time I was pregnant – partly because I wasn't married, and partly because of the HIV. He couldn't cope and he said that I was throwing my life away, and my boyfriend wasn't good enough. My dad is someone who can't face ugliness.

'HIV has changed my life completely – with it I've been through the worst of times and it's been like a massive wound.

'I visualized my situation as a big long black tunnel with no light at the end of it. I've now split up with my partner, although we are the best of friends. We've gone in different directions to deal with things – I've focused on therapy and rebuilding, but he wants to hide and has retreated into despair.

'He's threatened suicide. If we hadn't split up I feel like I would have died – I was totally drained from watching him destroy himself, watching him suffer, wallow in self-hate and feeling very alone.

'But there have been positive things – it's forced us to talk. Like with sex, before for me it was something that happened with the light out and you didn't talk about it, but now you have to put the light on and put the condom on.

'HIV has opened up our relationship a lot making us look at the things that are important – especially honesty. Now we don't hold back at all and the relationship is better partly because there is space to reach out. We are part of each other's make-up, especially because we went through adolescence together, and as I felt guilt and he has a neediness, we hooked into each other.

'The thought of death turns you upside down. When someone close to you is dying, it's a gaping wound that is always raw and you can't shut it off. It's important to resolve things so that you aren't left with ghosts.

'He got a letter from the hospital asking him to come in for a T-cell count – he doesn't want to live for dying and doesn't want to watch his health disintegrating. Our daughter is the most important thing he has and he sees us as a family. She has cushioned things for him. He has used a lot emotional blackmail, he uses it to get at me, taking advantage of my guilty feelings, and trying to get away with murder. It's important to work it all through. Sometimes there's the black tunnel – oblivion – which is like falling into a well, deeper and deeper, feeling that you'll never get out, but then, when you do come out the other side, it's the most releasing thing.

'I've gone beyond the fear of death. My first experience of finding out was a feeling that the present and the future had been taken away, I felt a blob . . . but now there's the excitement of being able to work through things and there's an oozing of light – a feeling of being free – deep joy and contentment.'

R

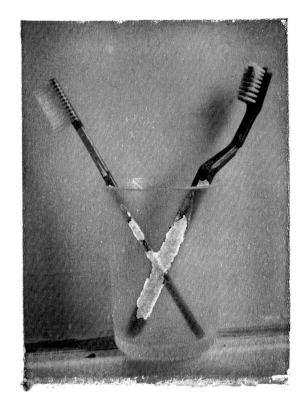

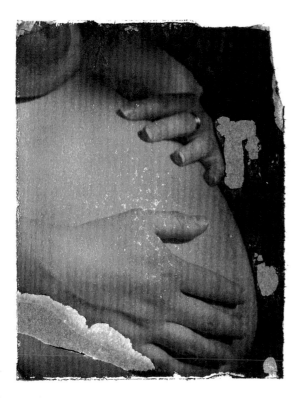

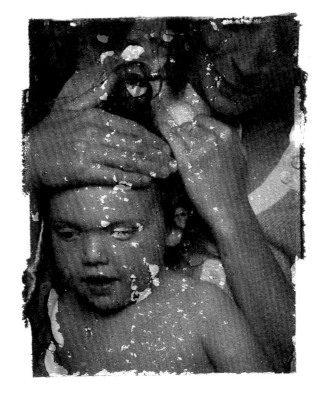

CHAPTER 8

RUPERT – A Life Story

Photographs by Paul Reas

'They called me up from the Terrence Higgins Trust and asked if I'd be interested to work with a photographer on a project about someone who has AIDS. The someone was me and the photographer was a man from Bradford. I must have sounded doubtful; they tried to encourage me by saying "Meet him anyway".

'So we met. Me and this northerner with a northern accent, sitting in my London kitchen drinking mugs of tea. He wanted me to tell him all about myself. I was wondering where to begin.

'My earliest childhood memory is of having my photograph taken. My mother perched my brother and me on a fallen tree a few yards from our house and took a snap that we still have in the family album. I told the man in my kitchen about that.

'But what I didn't tell him was that in the market that morning the stallholders had shouted out "AIDS!" as I walked by. Nor did I tell him what I had felt in the hospital three-and-a-half years ago when they told me that I had AIDS. Like tens of thousands of other gay men, the incubus had been sitting on my shoulder for a long time; with me fearing and dreading that one day it would be my turn. When at last it was, I sighed with relief.

'It is not the dying, nor the discomfort, it is the saying goodbye that is so hard. There's a German nurse at the hospital who has the tact of a sledge-hammer, but I like her. At the regular Monday morning clinic the other day, she said to me, "It's amazing that you are so well and everybody else is dead!"

'My mother wants lists of things in the house that are mine; friends worry that I haven't finalized my will; I talk to the priest about funerals; I've made arrangements for the dog; and now there's a guy in my kitchen asking me to tell me about my life.

'We drank more tea and he asked me if I'd make a list of all the places which are special or important in my life; the farm where we'd lived, bike rides with my brother, my school, the first gay bar, the cottage where I first got picked up.

'When he'd gone, I tried to imagine the photos he might take. The restaurant where I'd met my lover, the staircase to Bob's apartment in New York. Secret places, some of them places that I hadn't seen in twenty years. The house where my mother and father had their terrible rows, the blue square of carpet where I'd stood on my first day at school. Places that still haunted me . . . were these places still haunted by memories of me just as I am haunted by memories of them?

'It's a curious thing, but as you approach the end of your life, ambition and future plans give way to a need to remember. Like an old person I reminisce. I look back, sometimes shocked and even horrified, sometimes I laugh, remembering with embarrassment the things that I said, thinking of places and events not thought of for years. So it was that I sat down to write the list.

'A few days later in a pub in Covent Garden I handed it to Paul. A scrappy piece of paper, my life, summed up on a side of A4. It was clear that he would never find the locations mentioned on the list without me there to show him, and so on a sunny morning in May the two of us drove back to my childhood.

'On the way in the car I asked about the photos he planned to take. He said that they might be no more than suggestions of places and that he wanted them to be ambiguous, perhaps even abstract. I asked if I would recognize them; my school, the stream that my brother and I used to dam. He thought I might not, but I do, I recognize them all.'

Rupert Haselden

RUPERT'S ANECDOTES

Country Childhood

Myxomatosis spread through the rabbit population, across the neighbouring farms until eventually it was on our land. We were disgusted by 'mixy' rabbits. I remember how cross my uncle was when I wasted a shotgun cartridge on a sick rabbit. I should have killed it by stamping on it with my heel.

I was thirteen, lying in bed one night when I first said to myself, 'You are homosexual'. I remember thinking that it made me special. I remember being pleased and I was sure that it would lead to an exciting life.

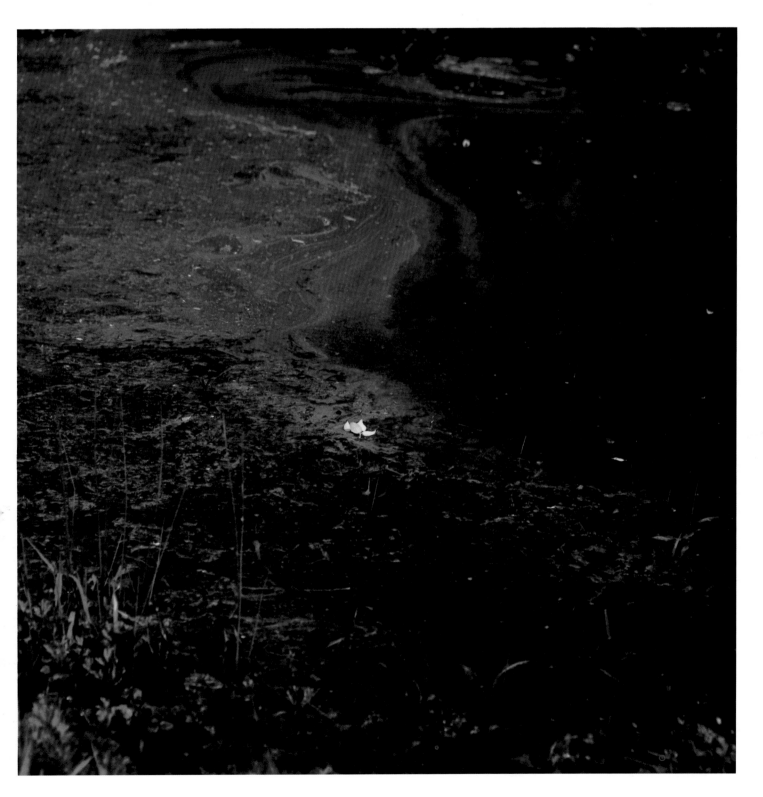

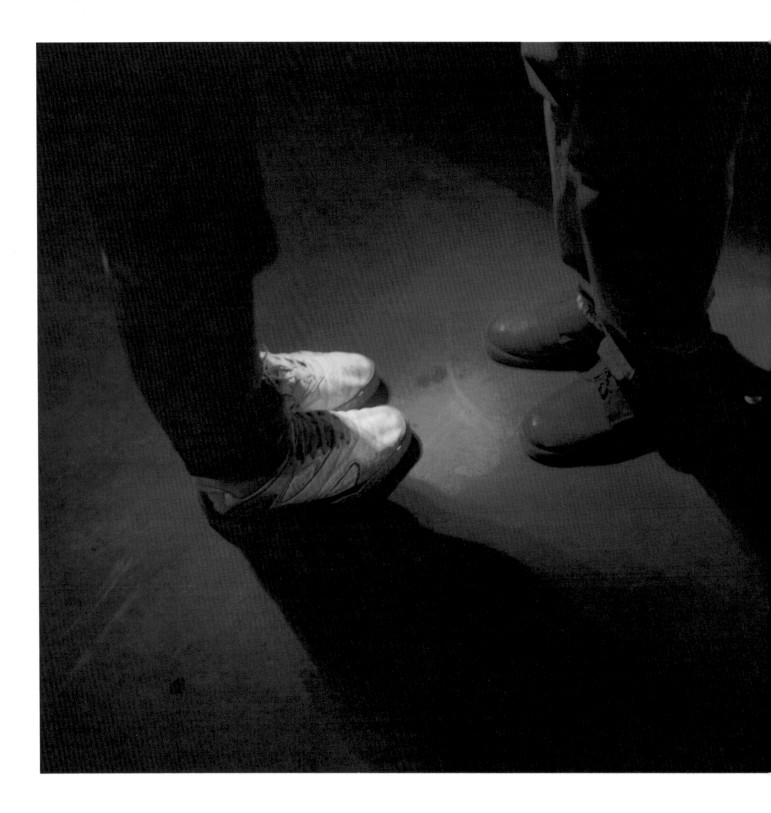

London

I had discovered that toilets were the place to meet people and so one day I followed a guy out of Piccadilly underground. He was about my age, perhaps fifteen. Aware of being followed he turned and looked at me.

'Are you rent?' he asked. Thinking that this must be slang for asking if I was queer I said, yes.

'Then there's no way is there, cos so am I,' he said. This left me very confused. Then, taking pity on me, he took me for coffee at Swan and Edgars and told me all about the gay scene.

For eight years I worked for Columbia Pictures. A large part of my job involved eating lunches in expensive restaurants. One day I was to have lunch with a BBC documentary director. He arrived late unloading crash helmets, carrier bags and leathers onto the restaurant floor. When at last he sat down he took one look at me and roared with laughter. He laughed so much and for so long that he only stopped when he hit his head on the wall behind him. A 23-year-old English public schoolboy was not his idea of a Hollywood mogul. We have now been lovers for twelve years.

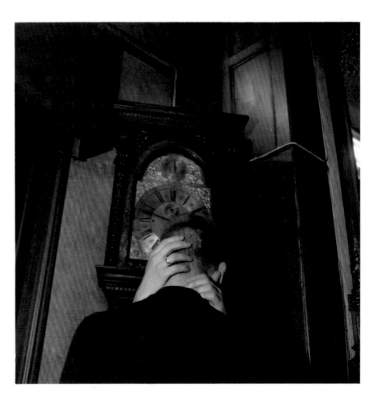

New York

We all wanted to go to New York and in 1978 it seemed like the only sensible thing to do. I was twenty and having a ball. On my second night I was taken to the bathhouse. I had never imagined so many good-looking men so freely available and I thought it was brilliant. As we left they offered us penicillin shots. I never did get clap in New York.

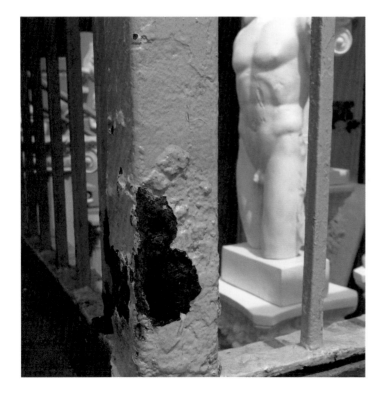

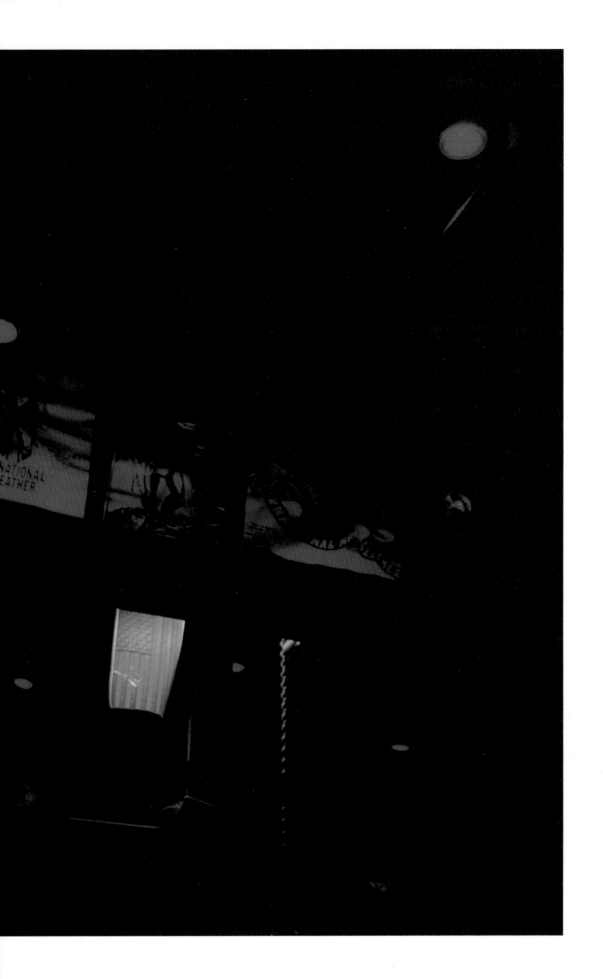

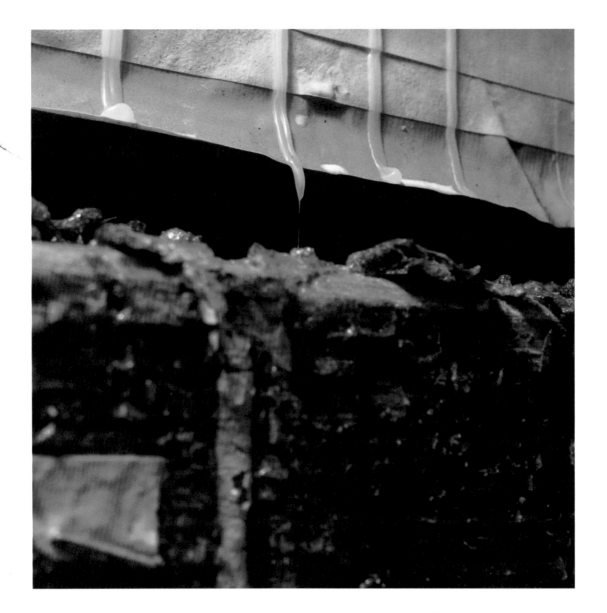

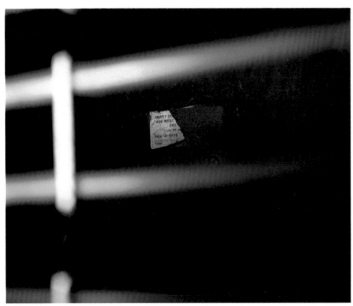

Bob's apartment was at the top of a long staircase. I would run up two at a time. It was the most glamorous apartment that I had ever seen. Like the rest of Bob's life it seemed to belong to the world of colour magazines. I have always thought that it was there in Bob's flat that I got HIV. I was back in New York not long ago and thought about climbing the stairs and asking whoever lives there now if I could see in, but I realized that I would never make it to the top. These days I'm out of breath brushing my teeth.

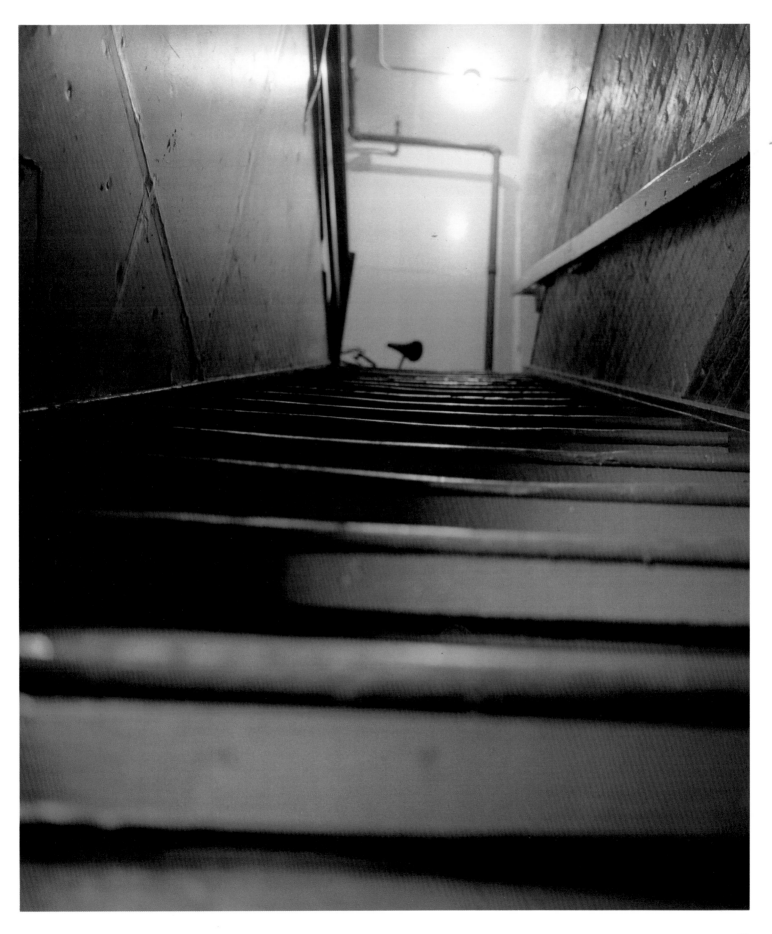

AIDS

My lover says I think too much about death and that he worries I've given up. I haven't, but I talk to a couple of priests, which I suppose in his book is tantamount to the same thing.

Along the side of my hospital notes is a row of little coloured stickers, like the stars given for good work at school. I have always felt that these stickers, one for each year of survival, are to be seen as a point of great pride. Currently I have five.

My sister's having a baby in a couple of weeks time and although no one has said it, I know that the whole family is terrified that I will get sick at the same time as the baby is being born. I hope I don't.

I hate the language that has grown up about AIDS, phrases like 'positive living' and 'PWA's'. When I became sick I was given a stack of books all with grisly titles like *Sharing the Pain*. People are very strange.

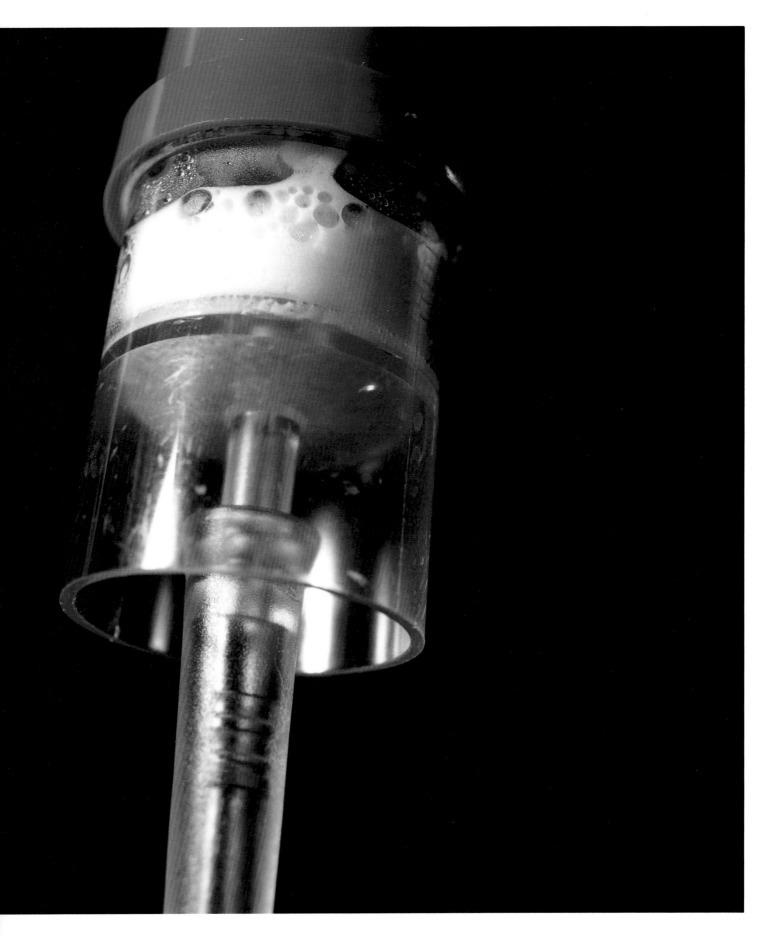

Home

My lover and I play a game which we've played for years.

He asks, 'When are you moving out?' and I tell him 'Probably very soon.'

'What will you be taking with you?' he asks, and I list all the things that I will be taking – the lawnmower, the big table, the carpets, the sofa without its cover, the drier that doesn't work.

A few months ago we invited a load of friends around for supper. I think that there were thirteen of us. Inevitably the subject of HIV came up when someone asked how many people around the table knew they were HIV-positive. Everyone except the person who had asked put up their hand.

I have a dog called Sam who I got from Battersea Dogs' Home eight years ago. I worry about what will happen to Sam.

My mother and I have recently been talking about things with a counsellor, a priest, one of those modern priests who says 'fuck'. I guess my mother is a modern mother too, because she also says 'fuck'. My lover tells our friends that she's a really interesting woman and I just think that she's brilliant.

My mother has now told almost all her friends that I have AIDS. I'm really glad she's told them. She says they've all been fantastic. We haven't told my grandmother yet, although we're planning to in the next few weeks.

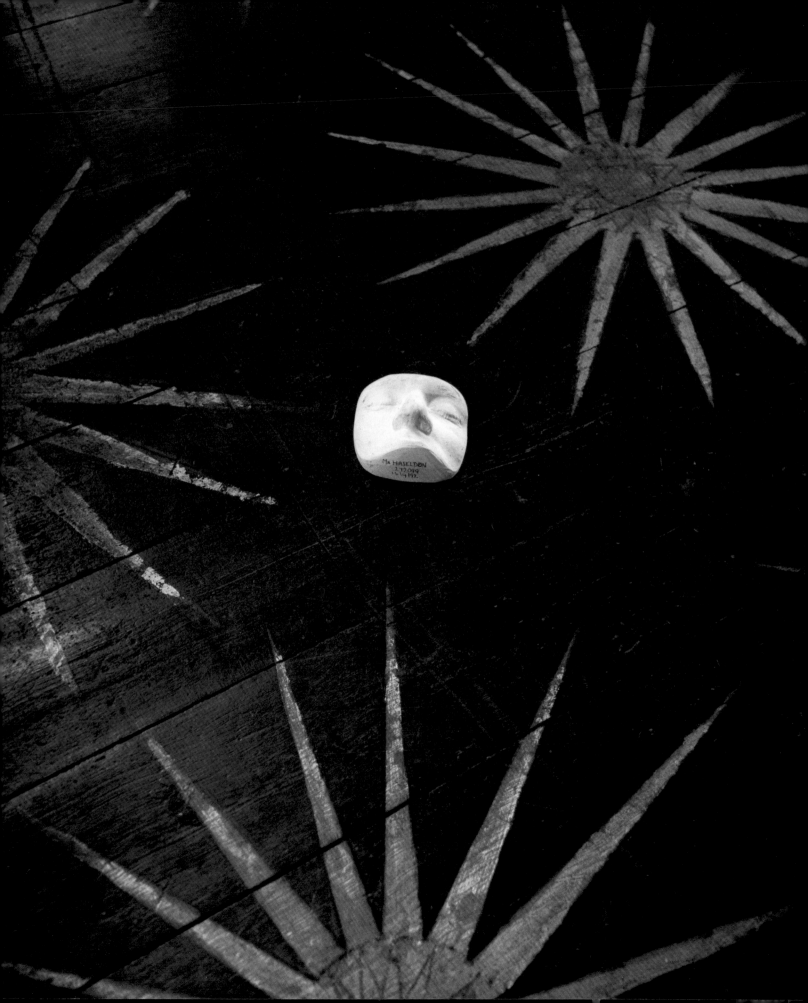

CHAPTER 9

GAY LIVES

Gay men have borne the brunt of the AIDS epidemic in Britain: not only the realities of HIV infection but also the epidemic of discrimination. We have been characterized as irresponsible and promiscuous and therefore undeserving of sympathy.

Despite continuing vilification, gay men have responded to the challenge of HIV and AIDS with dignity, responsibility and compassion. As a community we have created organizations which have informed, educated and cared for not only our own but everyone affected by the epidemic.

As individuals we have risen to the challenge of safer sex – celebrating different ways to be sexual adults, reflecting the diversity of ways we choose to live our lives.

Surely, rather than condemning gay men, shouldn't they be congratulated, thanked and supported for preventing the British AIDS epidemic from becoming a greater catastrophe than it already is?

Matt French

WINSTON

Photographs by Barry Lewis

Winston leads a wild life as a leading light at the London club 'Kinky Gerlinky'.

These pictures follow Winston through a night, revelling in the excitement of ambiguous social and sexual games, whilst his words demonstrate a highly developed sense of sexuality and identity.

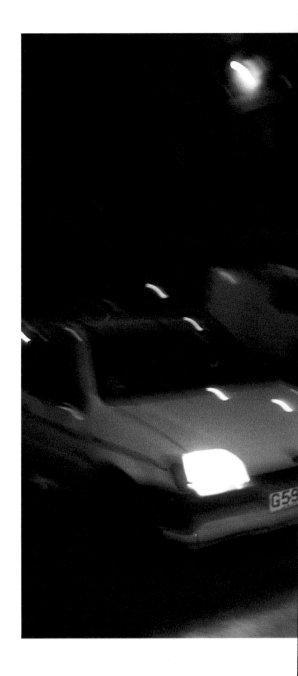

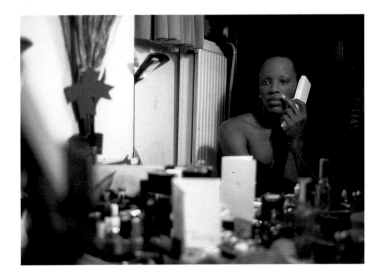

'People get off their heads for a few hours, but the reality is that problems never go away unless you do something positive about it. If we just decide to sit back and be negative about HIV and think we'll die anyway, we might just as well all run in front of buses or commit suicide. If you think that way, it's the end of your life.'

'People pigeonhole you to make themselves feel safe: "You're black, you're white" etc. Then they think that they know you.'

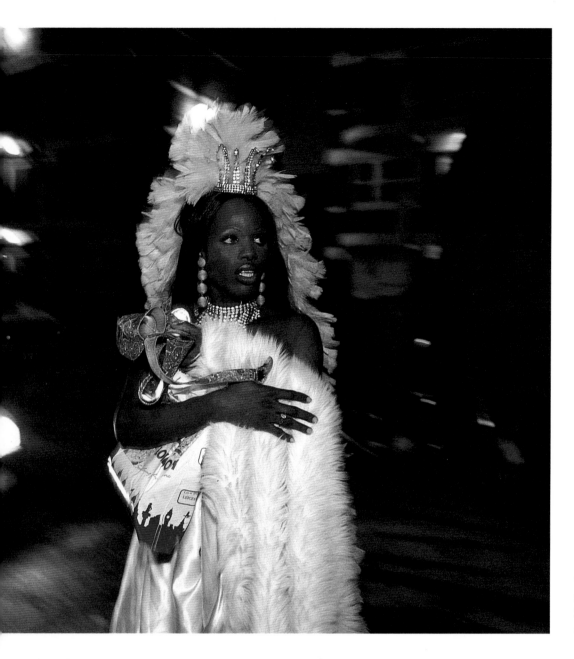

'What I do is about fun. There are times when you feel a bit lonely, you feel a bit miserable and you need company – it's those times when you need to look at yourself more closely. I try to do something positive: I create an excitement and an enjoyment from this whole depressing thing.'

'I'm going to have to face up to dying, but before that I want to find out how much living I can do.'

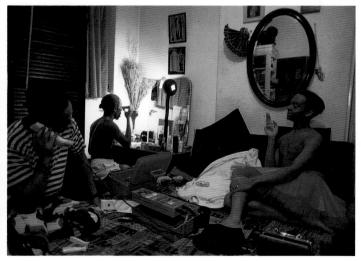

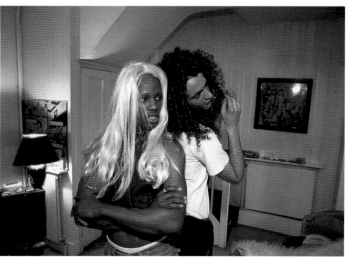

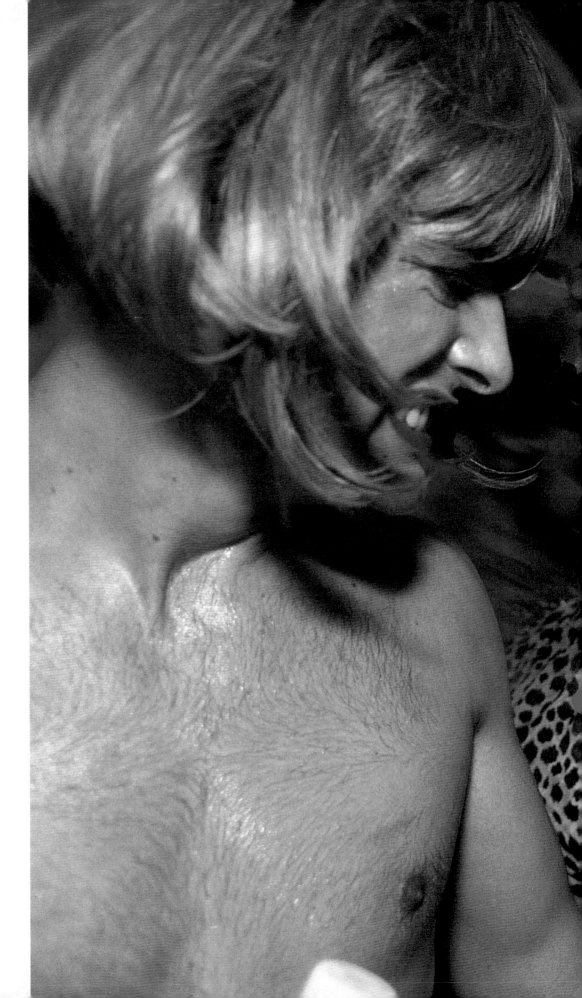

'People see being sexual as something freaky, something not to be mentioned, not to be touched, not to be played with.'

100

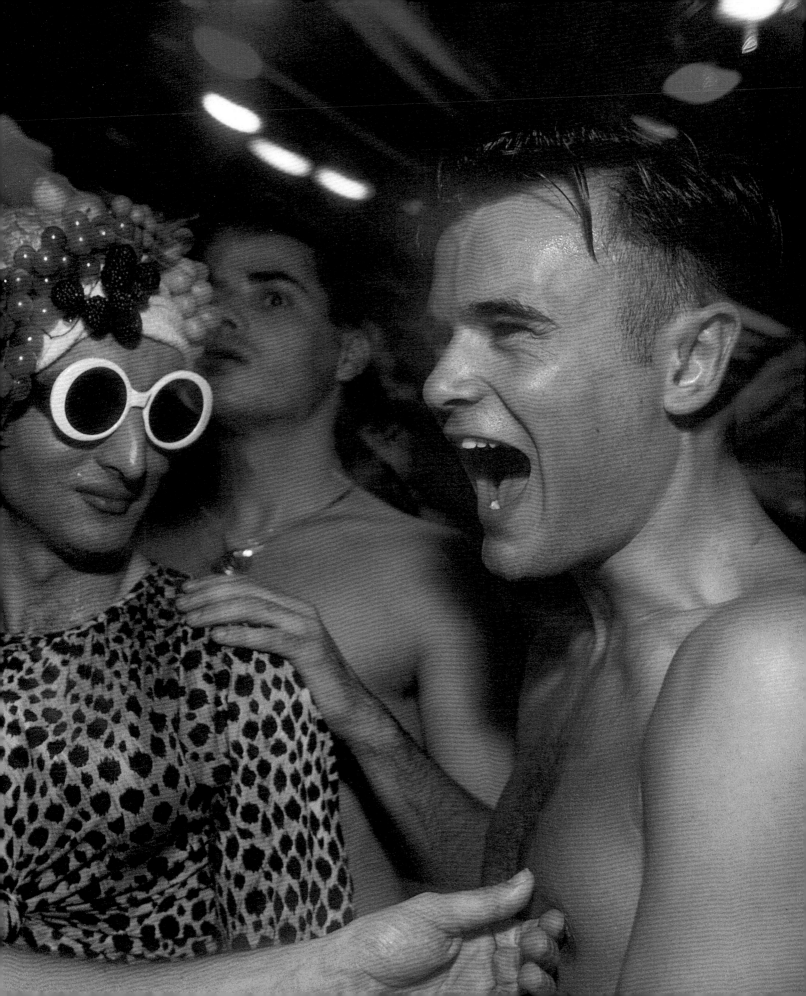

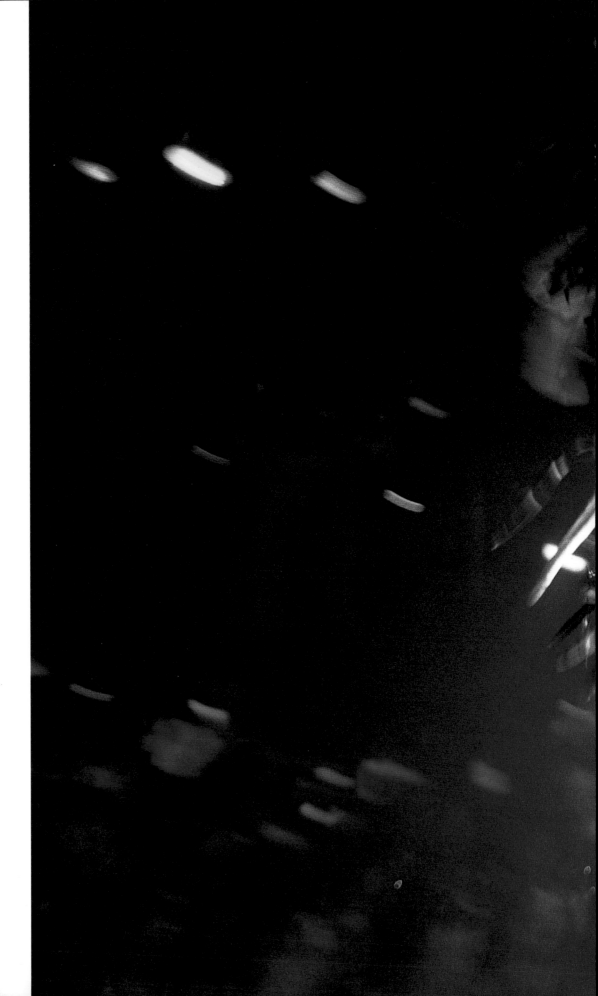

'I am fulfilled on a daily basis –
sometimes I'm broke and
sometimes I'm depressed, but
every day I have another chance.
For some people, when they are
ill, they count every day as one
day less in their lives – for me it's
one day more. It's an addition as
opposed to a subtraction.'

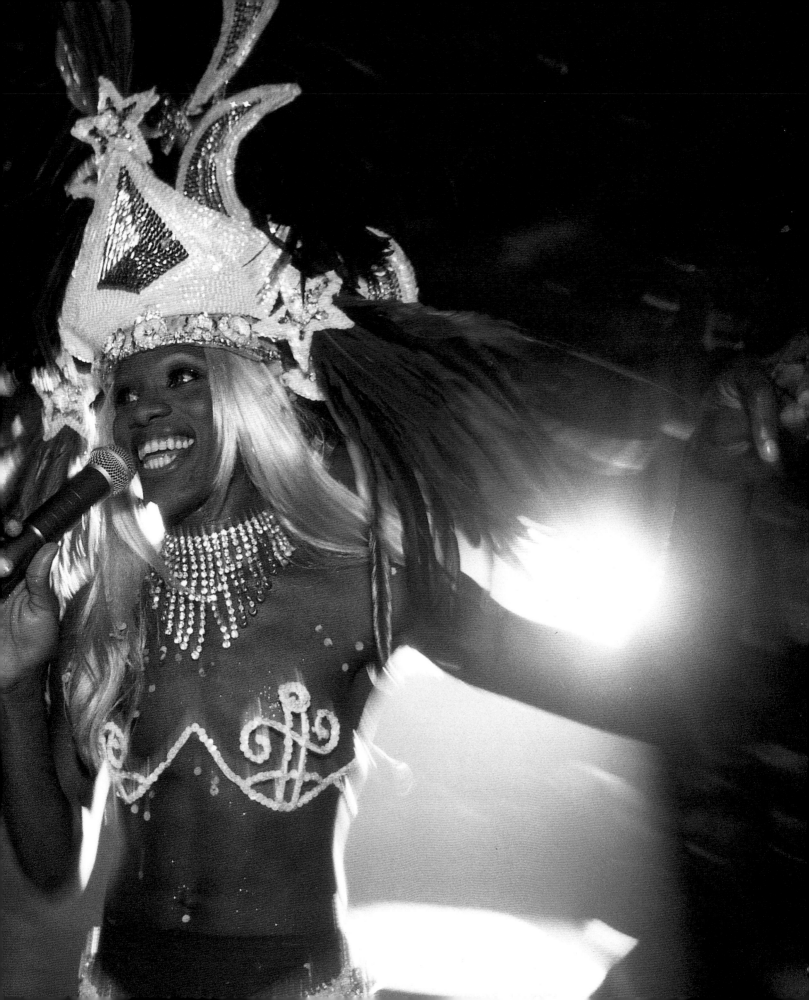

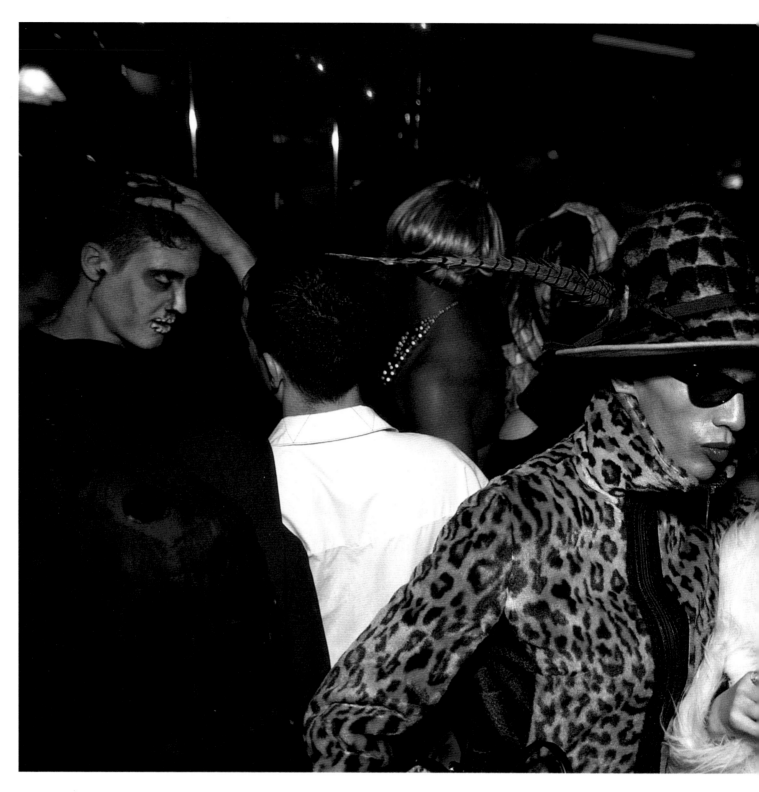

'Now with HIV around there are so many people dying of AIDS: they are friends of mine, friends of yours and friends of someone who has passed on because of it. But there is still so much life to celebrate. So many people around us get the attitude that they must give up – it's a hard thing to live with, but it doesn't necessarily mean that you have to go out and be an absolute slut without thinking about what happens tomorrow. Everyone should try to channel their energies into doing things that they consider healthy and positive.'

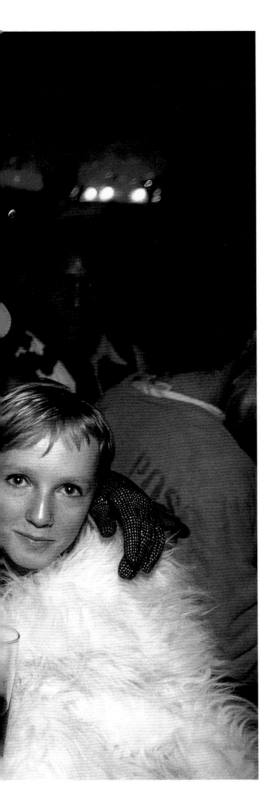

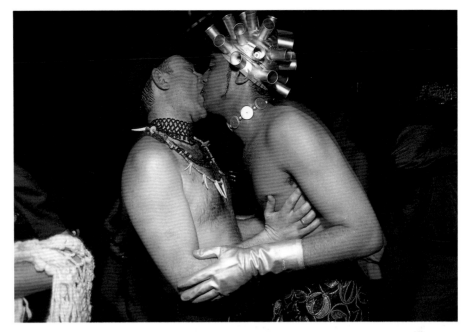

'I live every day like it's my last. I can imagine how devastating it is to be diagnosed HIV – you must live, don't just say "We have to die anyway". What's the point of dying if you haven't lived?'

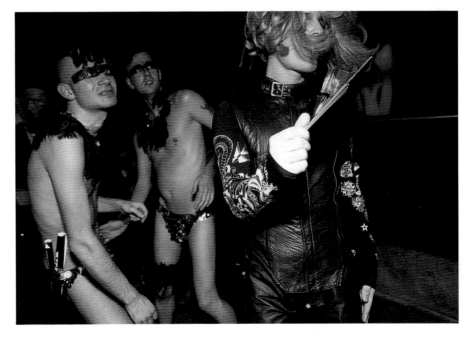

'Be careful what you do – you have to live with the repercussions.'

At least we had warning.

In 1981, AIDS had already established a silent, secure hold in the USA when the early cases appeared in clusters amongst gay communities in New York and San Francisco. Researchers were soon saying confidently that the illness was caused by a virus. If they were right, it was quite likely that the virus would cross the Atlantic.

First off the mark in Britain was the gay press which had learned a lesson from the US press. Slow to pick up the story, the papers there forfeited the confidence of their readers, making it harder later to pass on crucial information about the disease and its transmission. British papers got in early and unsensationally, so that readers were able confidently to weather the storm of lurid misinformation served up later – much later – by the tabloids.

Up until 1983, a serious attitude to AIDS in Britain was the exclusive preserve of lesbians and gay men. The first conference on AIDS was organized not by the National Health Service but by London Lesbian and Gay Switchboard. The first doctors in the field, many of them gay, read the gay press for their information; there was nothing for them in medical journals (the Oxford English Dictionary credits *Capital Gay*, a free weekly newspaper, with the first use of the term 'HIV'; second was the international science journal *Nature*). When the Terrence Higgins Trust was launched by three gay friends, its first funding came from collection tins rattled at benefit drag nights in London pubs.

In a strange reversal of roles, patients became the experts in their disease whilst the doctors were still learning, forcing the medical profession to rethink the role of patients in their own treatment – a fundamental re-evaluation that has since extended beyond the field of AIDS and which many doctors and nursing staff have now come to welcome.

In the eyes of gay men, 'people' were falling ill and dying. But when newspaper editors and policy makers finally turned their attention to the disease, they saw 'only homosexuals' as being affected. 'No cause for alarm', they reassured the heterosexual master race. In their confusion, AIDS appeared to be merely a component of a broader sexual pathology – namely homosexuality. They dubbed it 'the gay plague', blissfully and deliberately ambiguous as to whether gay men were suffering from a plague or whether gay men were, in themselves, the plague.

In the gay community frustration mounted as it became increasingly clear from the American experience that heterosexuals too could develop AIDS. Ironically, it seemed that the homophobia which was stopping the Government and the press from taking AIDS seriously meant that heterosexuals would pay with their lives this time, not just gays. If anyone took grim satisfaction from that, it must have been tempered by the further reflection that it would always be the under-privileged who paid.

When the message finally got through, the public information campaign that ensued was aimed not at gay men in the front line but at heterosexuals.

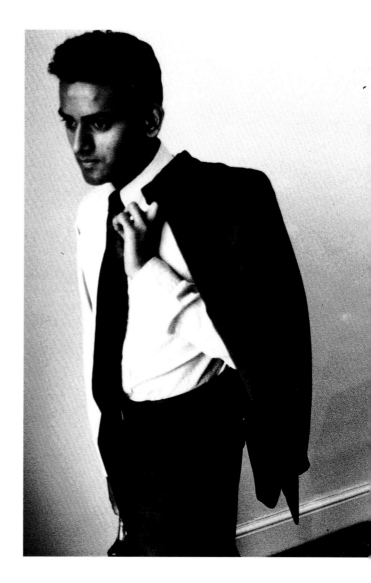

This time the old message has finally got through – it's self-reliance or die. The way ahead is now pointed by organizations like Gay Men Fighting AIDS, local gay outreach projects, and special interest groups like SM gays who rejoice in the well-earned reputation which gay men have for sexual generosity, and aim to foster a nationwide popular safer-sex movement, whilst campaigning to protect welfare services for PWA's from a cuts-mad government.

Michael Mason

AAMIR AND MARTIN

Photographs by Christopher Pillitz

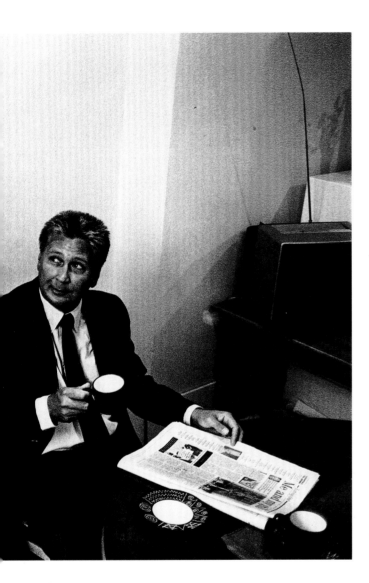

This is a gay plague.

A plague of hatred, prejudice and intolerance spread against the gay community. While we've been creating our own support groups, educating ourselves and funding our carers, the media have been making criminals out of the victims. While we've been fighting for money that we need, that we have paid in taxes, the authorities have been too busy trying to decide whether straights are affected so as to justify any expenditure. The fact that people are dying seems to be irrelevant if they're queer.

So if you don't like our lifestyles, you have no right to comment, because when we are dying or crying or grieving you are only there to add to the misery. Soon you may come to realize that we have long stopped caring what you think of us. We just want you out of our lives. If AIDS does spread to the general population, don't expect compassion in return for the scorn you gave us. We're not saints or angels, just people exhausted from years of supporting our own.

Our existence has been denied in the media, in public life and on the streets. So, we've defined ourselves and explored and understood our sexuality unaided. When we go cruising, we are saying that we are comfortable with sex, that we are not ashamed of it. Contrary to popular perception we are not driven by sex. If we were, we'd be easy to dismiss. Instead we are honest enough to allow the expression of our sexuality without letting it overwhelm us.

The two of us have been together for nearly ten years. Yet we do not pretend that we will never be attracted to another man. The strength of our relationship is that we can let our partner have sex with someone else. We don't need to have secret liaisons. We don't have to lie to each other. We know the relative importance of love and sexual fidelity.

Imagine if there were straight cruising grounds. At any time you could go to them and within five minutes find someone to have sex with. Think about it. How many people would not be tempted on their way home from work? How many would be close enough to their partners to admit it to them? For that matter how many husbands or wives would understand? Your relationships would be destroyed by simple honesty, whereas ours are deep enough to be strengthened by it.

So when you see images of us having sex, realize that by being open we are being honest to ourselves. That is our surest defence against the 'gay plague'.

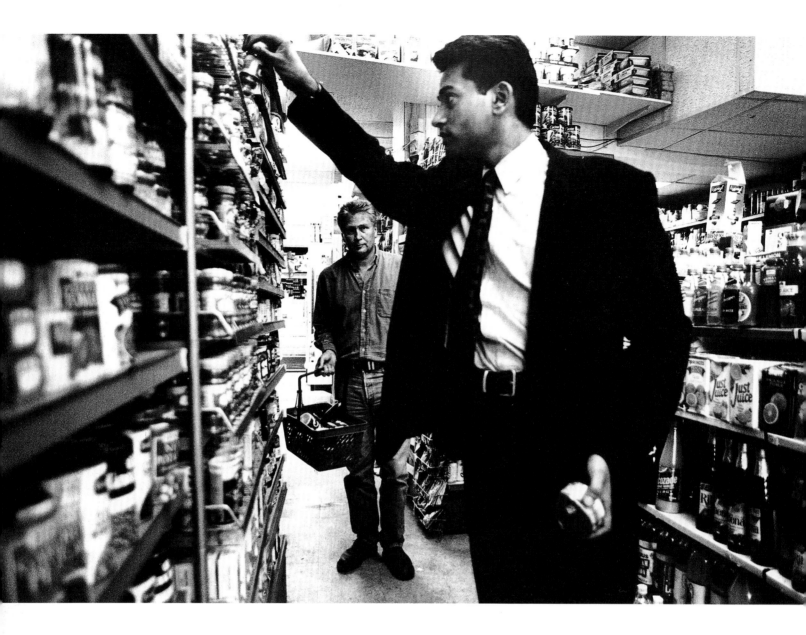

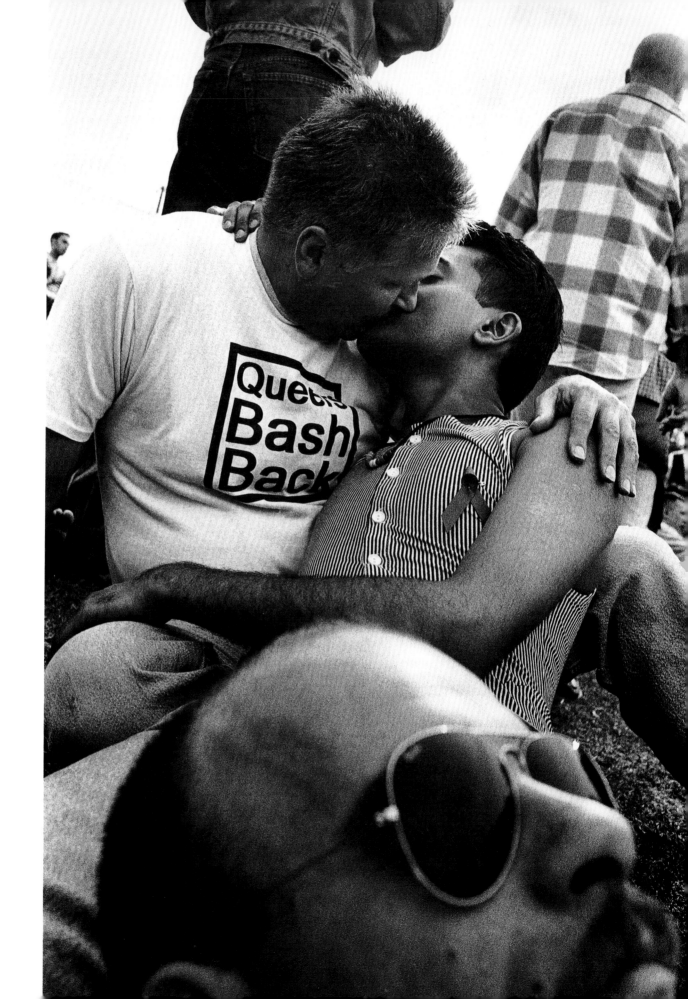

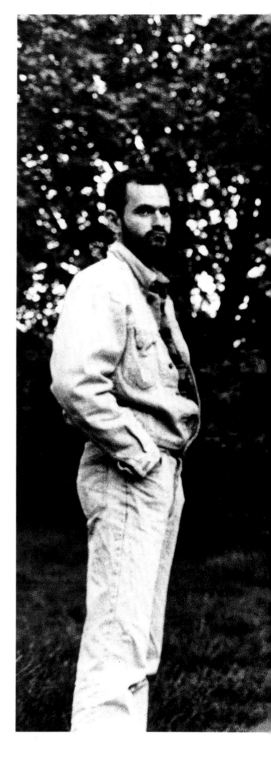

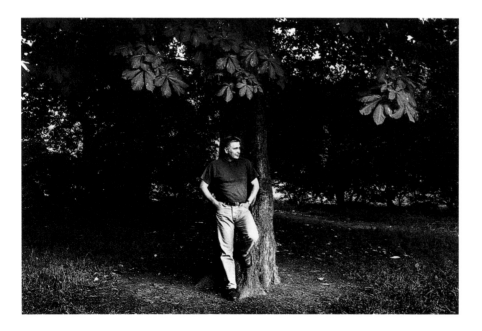

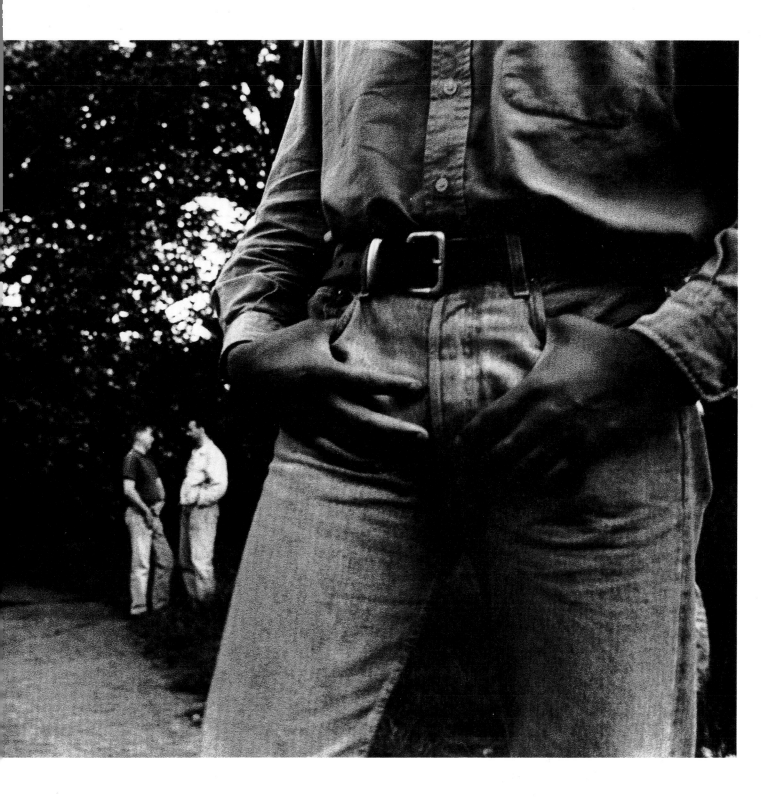

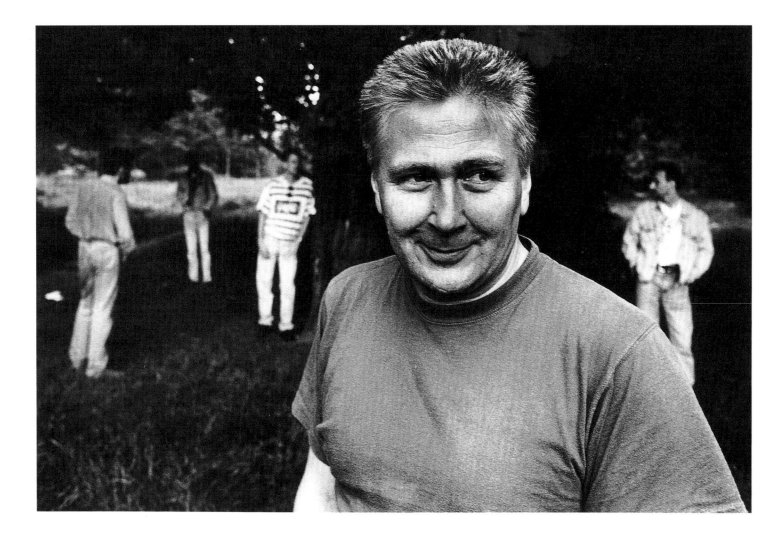

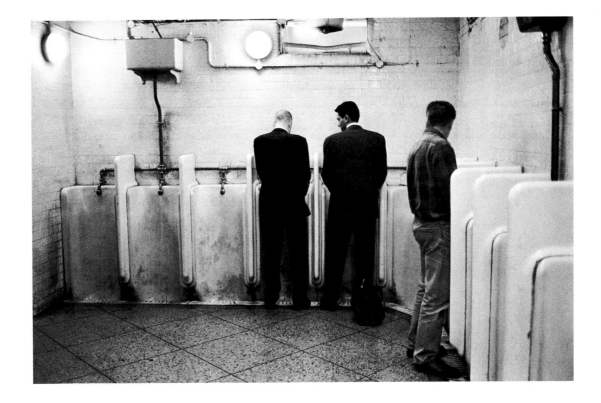

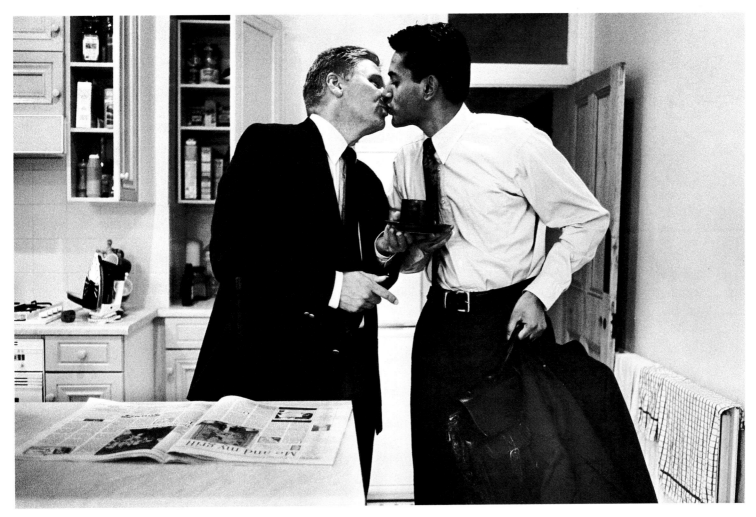

CHAPTER 10

SEX –
If Looks Could Kill

Photographs by Denis Doran

Power is at once threatening and an aphrodisiac. A fetish is a symbol of power; fetish sexuality is an empowering process. These photographs are of people who express their sexuality through fetishism, whether that fetish be a dog-collar or a string of pearls.

Power is also an expression of control. In the ritual of sado-masochism, this is manifested in a control over physical sensation and psychosexual experience. Within the tribalism of fetish culture, control is expressed through body decoration and dress.

Power is often confused with aggression. Fetishism, considered as literally and metaphorically dangerous, is seen as an outward expression of violence. But power-play is participation in a theatre of paradox, not of violence. Paradoxes exist within the dynamics of pleasure–pain, empowerment–enslavement, control–trust and danger–safety.

Power-play incorporates elements of danger but it is conducted within safe parameters, using safe words, safe thresholds and safe sex. These people may look dangerous, but they understand the importance of safety.

Pas Paschali

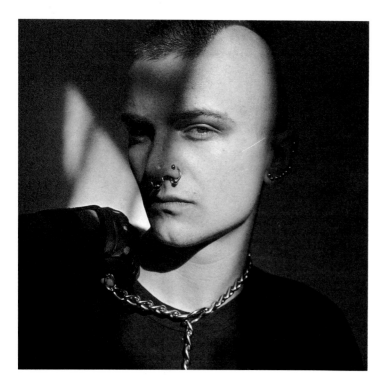

'Confront disability, sex, homosexuality and death – confront your fear. I did. I confess to pleasure and to safety. I'm not about to apologize for it.'

Gavin

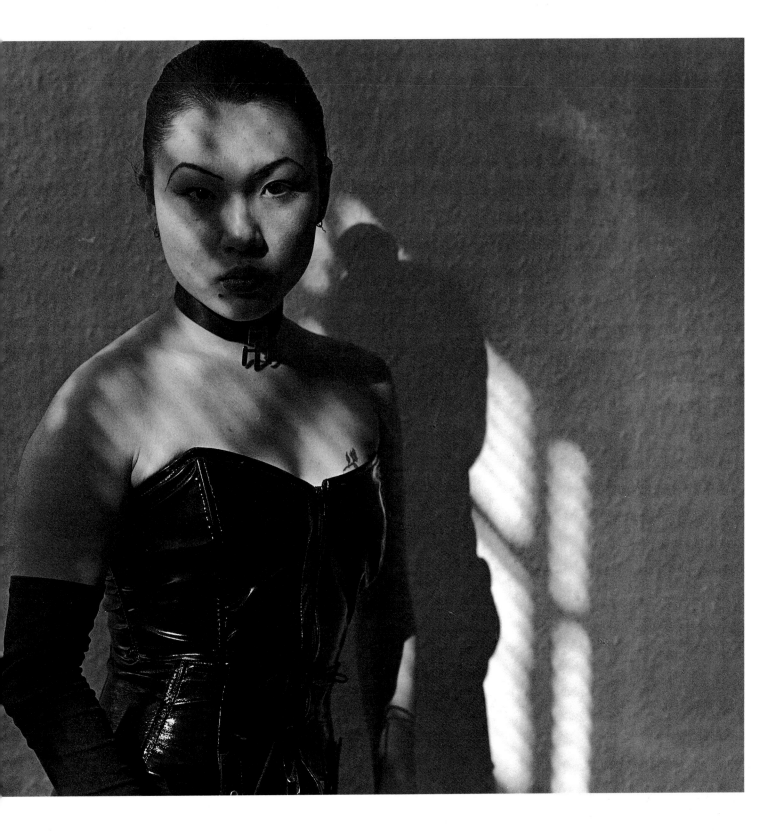

'I think that it is one of the principles of fetish dressing – the body must be cared for. If you put these clothes on a neglected body you end up looking pretty stupid!'

Koari

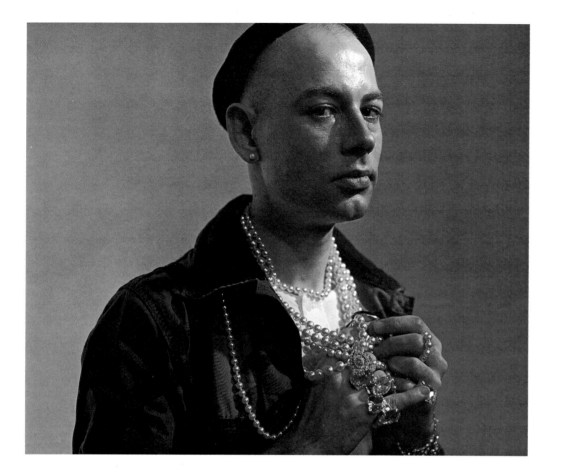

'The pearls? Everybody hates it when I wear my pearls with army fatigues, particularly in the gay bars. You see, there *my* appearance is expected to fulfil *their* sexual fantasies of machismo. The point here is that I know when I wear the right clothes, because for me it *is* sex.'

Robert

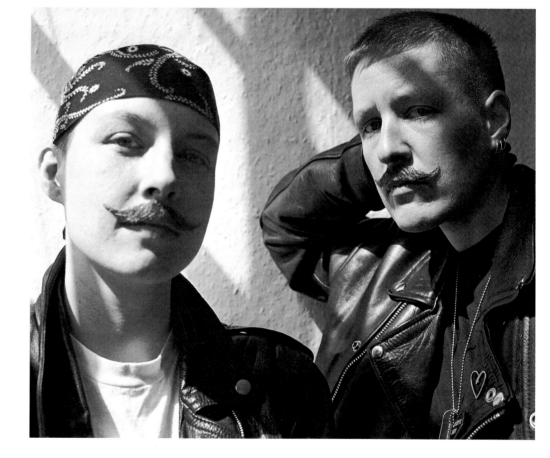

'People always want to know what we are – men or women, SM dykes or queer boys, drag kings or queens, transvestites or transsexuals. Somehow a label makes them feel safe. But listen, we like to push at the boundaries of gender and sex. The only thing that is safe about us is the way we play – sexually.'

'Hawk' and 'Boy Chick'

116

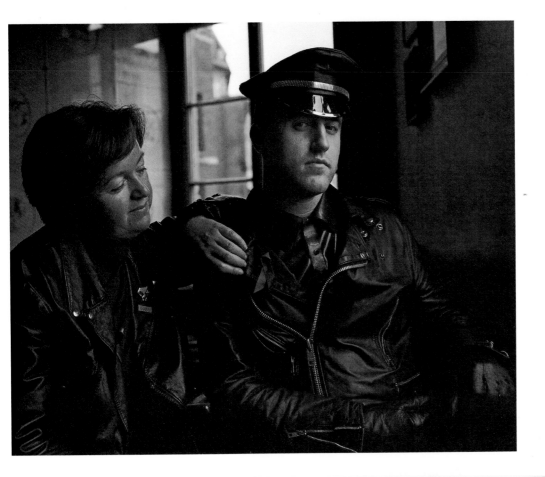

'Real families? Pretended families?
Show me the difference. But
about safe sex – they need to be
aware.'

Bonnie and Berkeley
(mother and son)

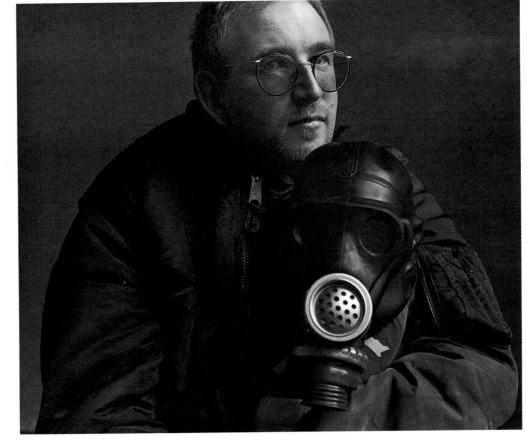

'All the world's a stage and all
men and women merely players;
some of them are safe and some
are not.'

Graeme

. . . of course I love metal – it's strength and power. I do my piercing when I feel strong and then I have control. And yes, I'm sure that some people do find me offensive, but then they also want to touch me! In the street, people have approached me and insulted me and then wanted to touch my nose and ears. It's foul!'

Fran

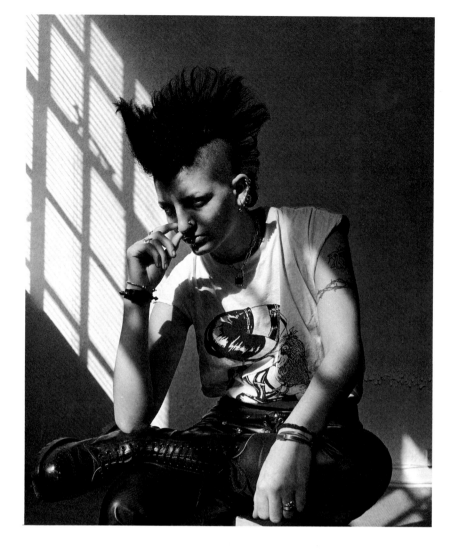

'Of course some people probably don't see me as a typical parent. But then I'm not quite sure what makes a typical parent. But this is quite clear to me, I want to be around to see Sebastian grow up.'

Charlotte and Sebastian
(mother and child)

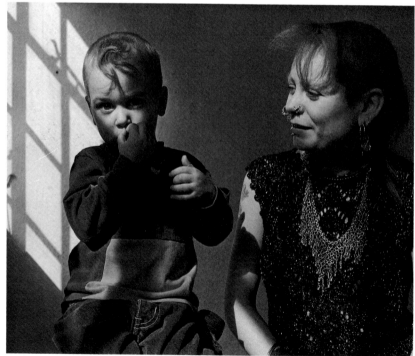

'Oh, I'm sure that some people do find the image offensive, but look at them! They may look "safe", be "sensible". But what of their sex practices? I'm safe – what about them?'

Cheimi and Koari

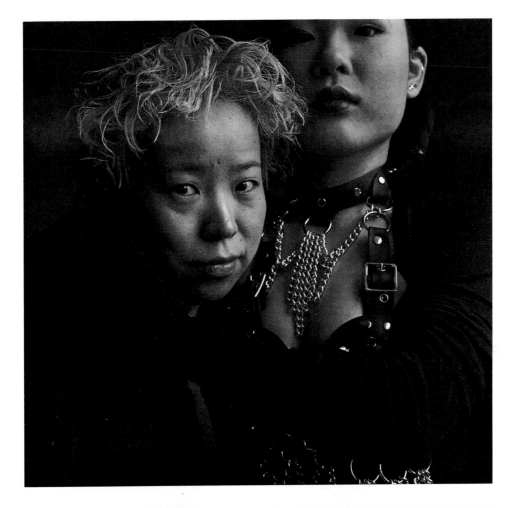

'It's not that we're ignorant or even immune to the publicity but it boils down to trust. We've been seeing each other for a long time now, on and off. We've both had other partners and we talk about it. We both assure each other that we had protected sex with the other partners and we have to believe each other. To start wearing condoms in our relationship now, at either person's request, undermines that trust – unfortunately, that's the risk.'

Jeremy and Tracy

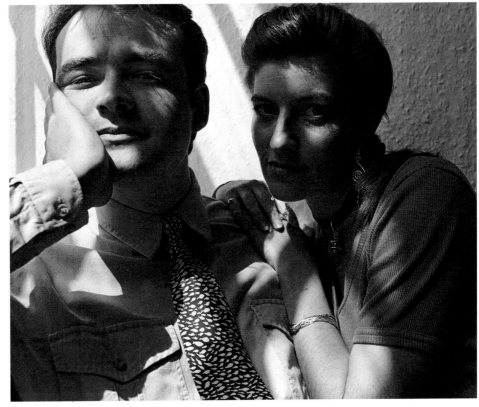

CHAPTER 11

ANOTHER VIEW

Photographs by Steve Pyke

Just as syphilis, TB and leprosy were once the objects of fear and ignorance, so today AIDS and HIV can evoke irrational and unsympathetic reactions.

From the first appearance of AIDS, effective prevention, treatment and support have been inhibited by misinformation and prejudice. Although things have improved in the last few years, there are still many people who refuse to acknowledge that this issue should concern us all.

The people portrayed here argue that AIDS and HIV is only a minority problem, one that does not deserve an urgent and compassionate response.

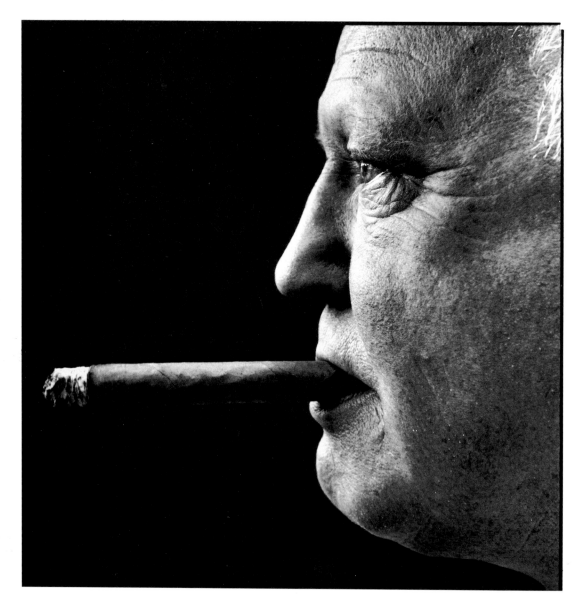

Brian Hitchen,
editor of the *Daily Star*

'How many families have been sentenced to death by faceless blood donors who were drug addicts or permissive homosexuals? And how long are we going to support spurious AIDS charities for those who brought this awful curse upon themselves?'

Daily Star

Sir John Junor,
Mail on Sunday columnist

'It is said that by shaking hands
with patients in an AIDS ward,
Princess Diana showed that the
disease need not make them into
social outcasts. But since each
had only his homosexual
promiscuity to blame for the
disease, isn't that exactly what
they should be?'

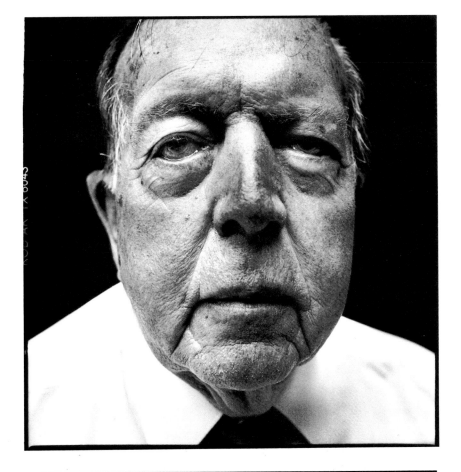

Stephen Green,
Chairman of the Conservative
Family Campaign

'A coalition of AIDS groups
produced a *Declaration of Rights of
People with AIDS* for launch in
1991. . . . So it was that they
demanded the right of people with
AIDS to all and any employment,
to mix with prisoners in gaols, to
sexual activity, including procre-
ation, and to much else that one
might think of as totally inappro-
priate.'

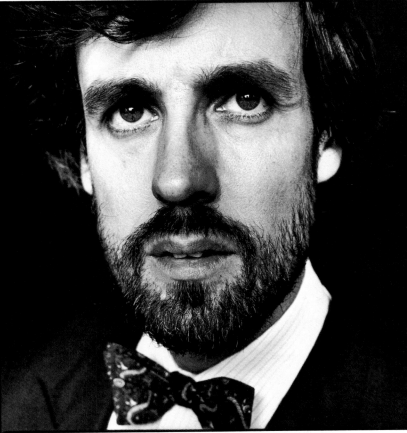

CHAPTER 12

CONSEQUENCES –
Acting It Out

Photographs by Paul Lowe

Growing up has never been easy. Today, voyages of sexual discovery have to be more carefully navigated than ever before. This project is a collaboration with the Theatre Royal Stratford East Youth Theatre Group in East London. The story was improvised by the actors and actresses, drawing on their experiences, hopes and fears, and shot in appropriate photo-romance style.

SACHA'S STORY

'So we were all at this party in my mate's house, you know, her parents were away and all that. Denise kept on saying to me, "He really fancies you, he keeps giving you the eye." So we started dancing together, and it felt really cool, like I was in control – he didn't make me feel scared or anything. Maybe I did flirt too much, but it felt good, no one discouraged me, they all kept egging me on. I didn't want it to stop and didn't want him to go home, at least not yet.

'Maybe I was too naïve, but I was loving it as much as him. I felt happy, comfortable – you can tell from the pictures that I was loving it! I didn't think we'd go all the way because I still felt in control, but then it all happened so fast that I didn't worry about anything else. I was only worried if he liked me.

'I wanted to see him again, if only to know that there wasn't a problem with AIDS. I got very upset – I was at breaking-point. Thinking about the night before, and all that had happened and all the problems that it caused the next day, I would have been more careful. If only I'd thought about the consequences I wouldn't have done it. I didn't even think about condoms or anything. It all happened too fast.

'He'd gone when I woke up the next day and I tried to tell myself that it was a dream. I felt rejected – he could have at least said goodbye. When I began to think about what might have happened next, I got really upset. I mean, I was in my friend's bed and who knows what he might have done. But I'd been getting some attention for the first time in months and it was great for a while, but really, was it all worth it?'

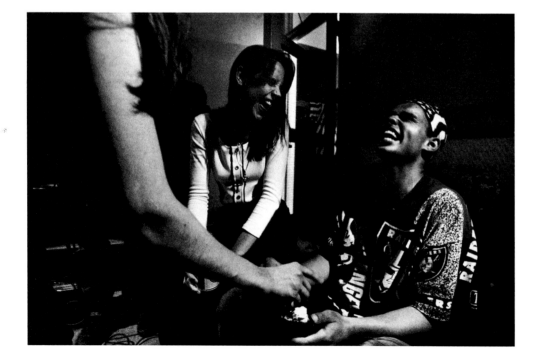

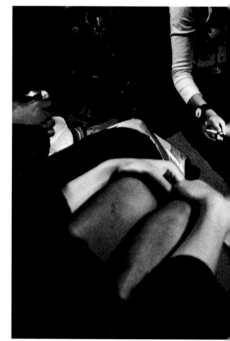

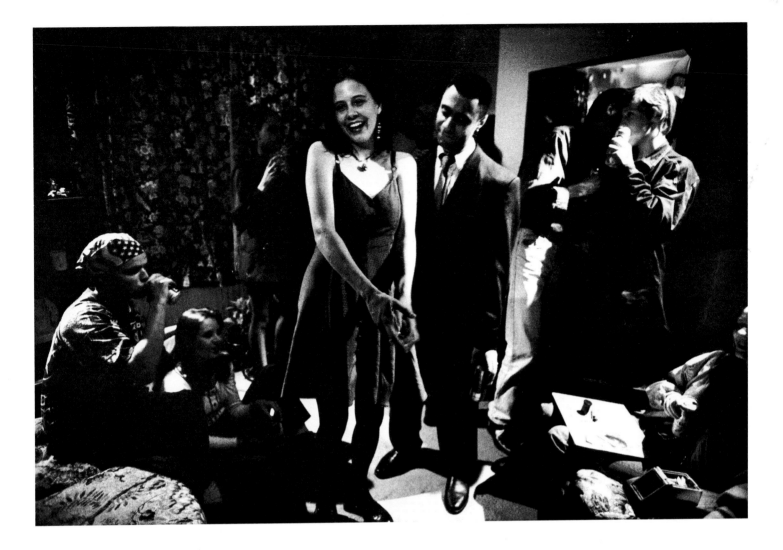

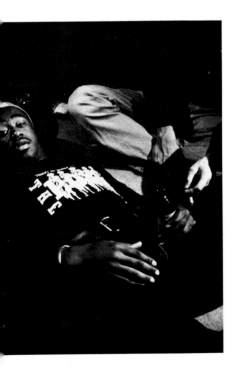

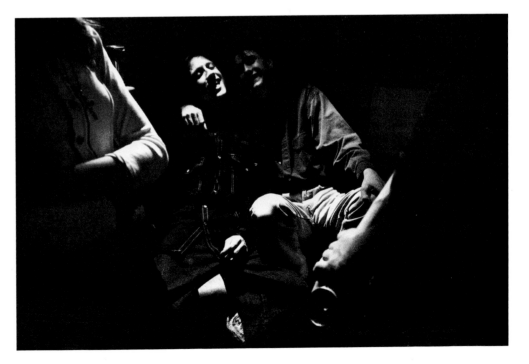

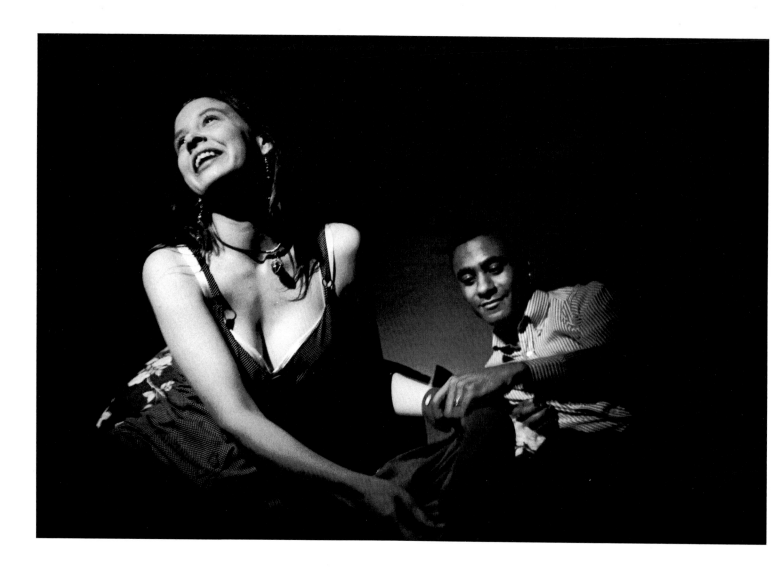

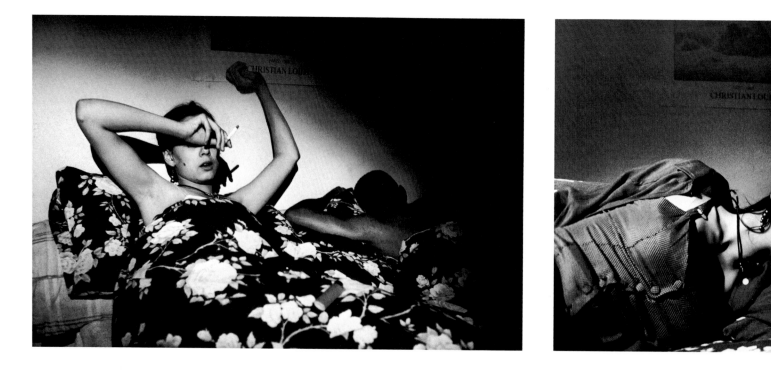

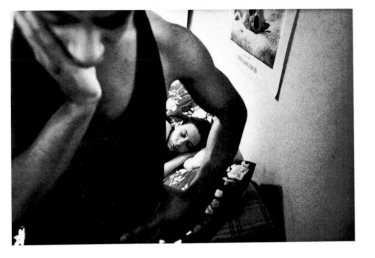

JOHN'S STORY

'Everywhere I went she was giving me the eye, so I thought I might as well have a go. No one at the party knew me, so I thought that I could get away with it. She even laughed at my jokes, so I knew it was going well, she knew what I was after. I didn't think of my missus, I suppose I'm a bit of a bastard really, only interested in one thing.

'In the cold light of day though, I had a massive hangover, and I thought, well she's a nice girl, she looked clean, but I've got to get home before my missus. I felt a bit guilty not saying goodbye, but it's less complicated like that, that's the way it goes really.

'Down the pub later, with all me mates, well, they were all pulling my leg, so I was boasting a bit about giving her one. But when she walked in and started shouting, I thought what's she going on about, she had a good time, what more did she want?

'It's a bit rough at home sometimes, but I love her really, but now she's pregnant, well I've got to have fun somewhere, haven't I? I mean, it's summertime.'

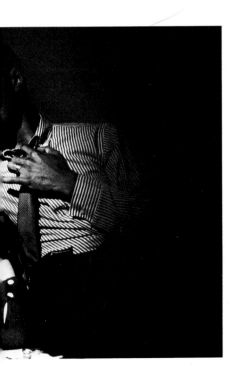

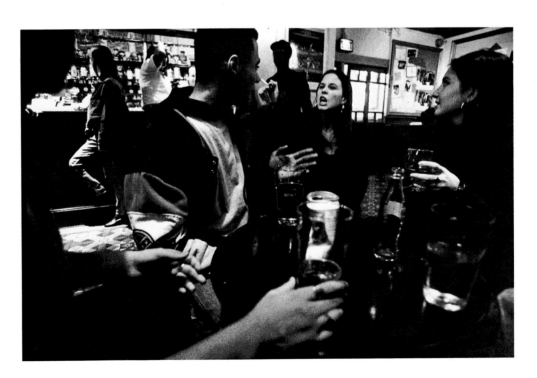

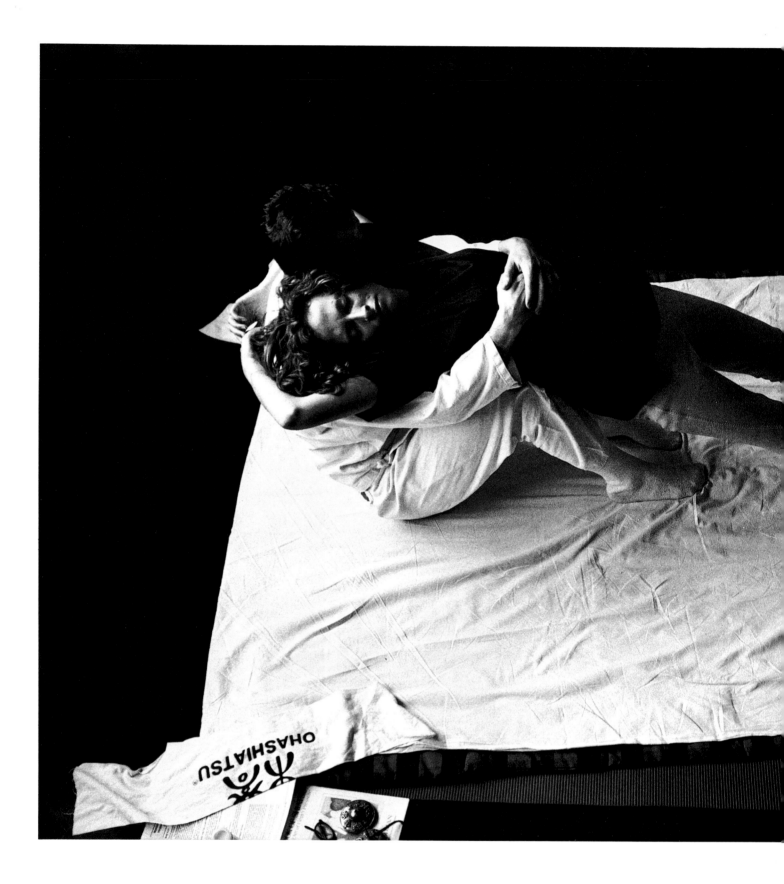

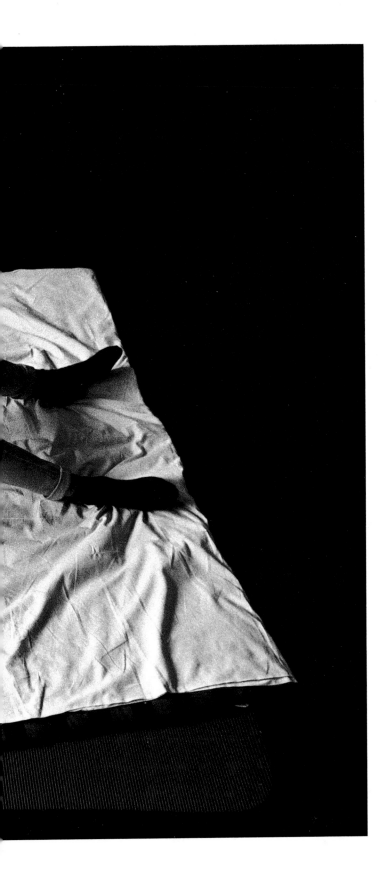

CHAPTER 13

THE WARDS

Photographs by Gideon Mendel

An AIDS ward is different. As the disease itself is so unpredictable and unusual, the treatment that has evolved is unlike any other. Although the latest in medical technology is being used, although constant new research is being carried out, the striking originality of AIDS treatment is in its approach to the needs and emotions of the patients.

These pictures at the Middlesex Hospital show some of the innovations that may prove influential in the treatment of other serious diseases. The staff, the patients, their friends and families work together in a way which we do not expect. Rather than being passive recipients of treatment, patients take an active role and are often extremely knowledgeable about their condition. Many are young, educated and articulate, and the wards have responded to their demands for control and co-operation. The staff, too, approach their work differently. They become attached to their patients, they can become their friends, and the friends of their friends and families. Often, when a patient dies, members of staff will attend the funeral.

AIDS is a changing disease, and as it changes further, so the wards will have to change. Although the majority of patients now are men, most of them gay, a steady trickle of female patients is appearing. These patients will have different needs, different demands. In a few years' time, perhaps, there will be a new revolution in treatment and a new perspective on disease and survival.

Shiatsu sessions are available, free of charge, for members of the hospital team who work in the AIDS wards, to help relieve some of the stress that results from working with people with AIDS every day. Shiatsu works on the principle that touching in a caring manner helps to trigger self-healing.

John

Since these pictures were taken, John has died. John showed remarkable fortitude and spirit during his illness, and the ward staff expressed great admiration for his courage.

He was in and out of the ward ever since it opened. On a number of occasions he chose to break off his treatment and go on holiday, and in his last year he travelled to Florida, Turkey and Spain, continuing his treatment on his return.

For John, his partner, his parents and friends, the ward became almost a home. His mother and lover would often sleep over at the hospital. Such informal images of life in a hospital ward would not have been possible even a few years ago.

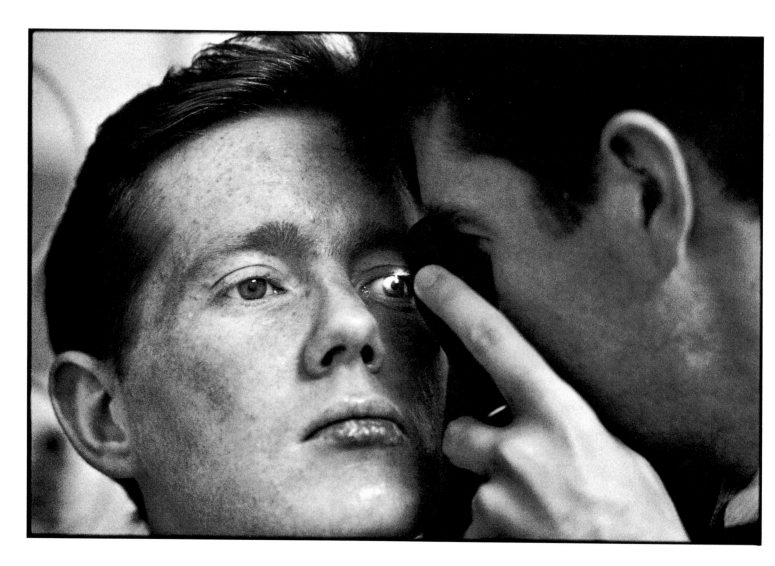

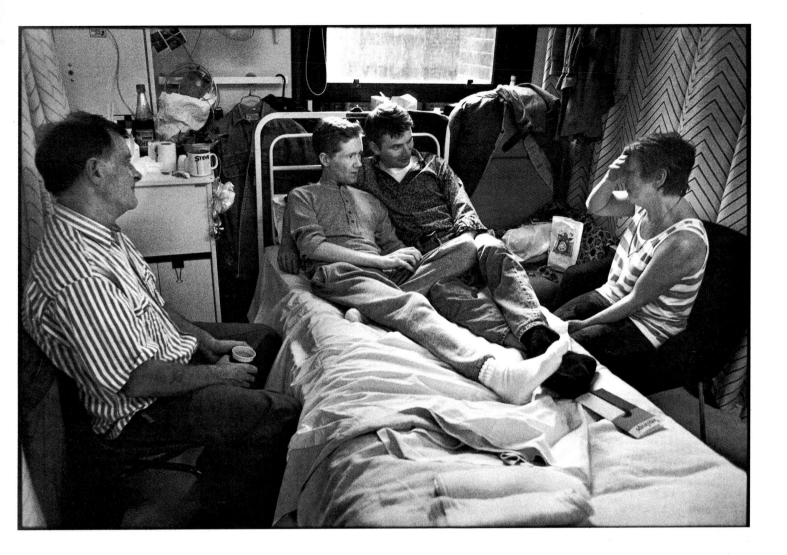

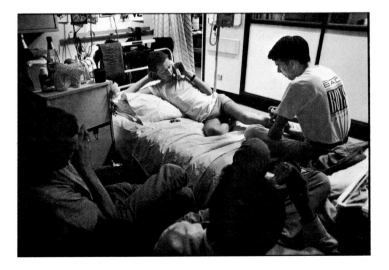

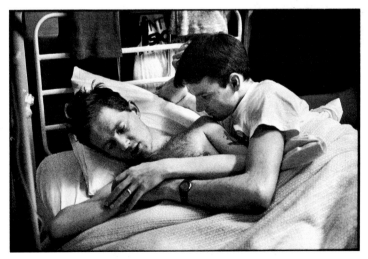

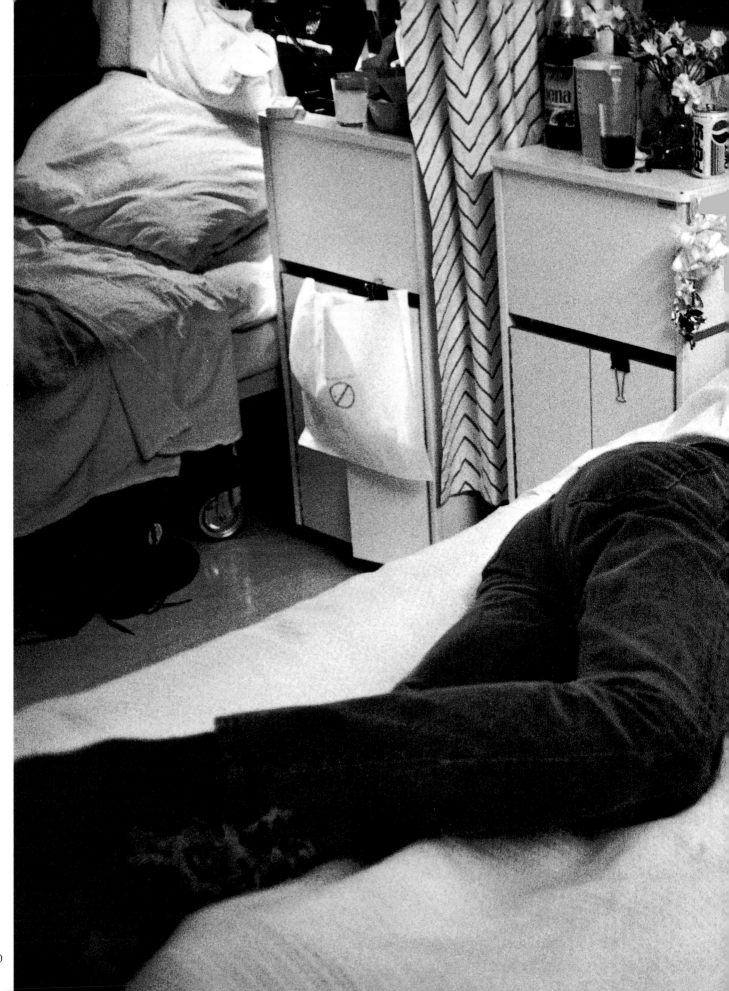

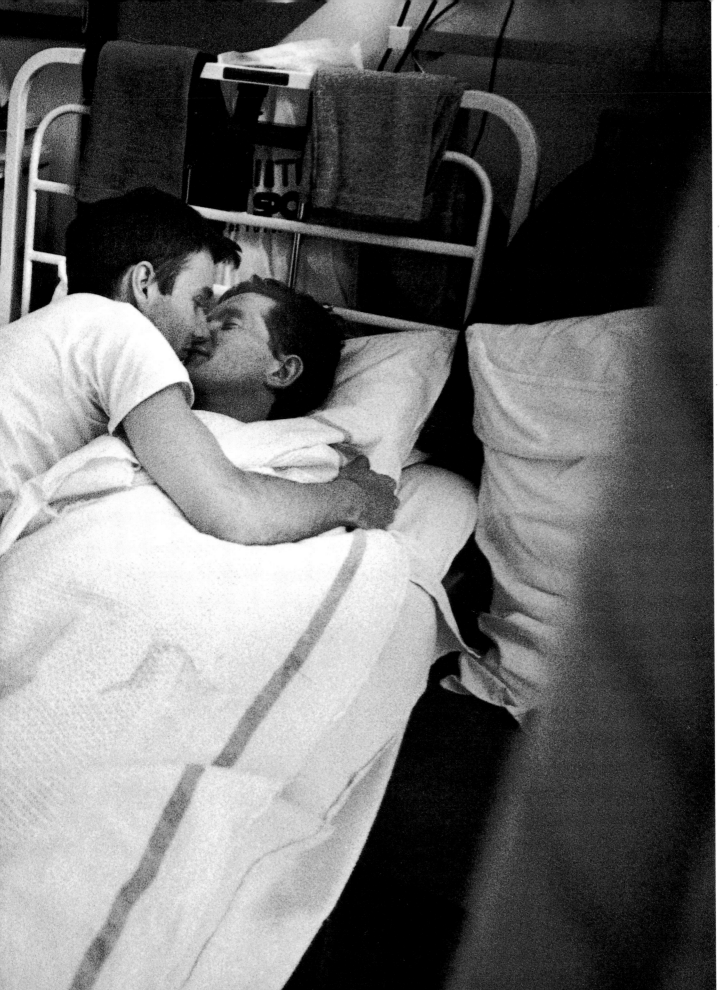

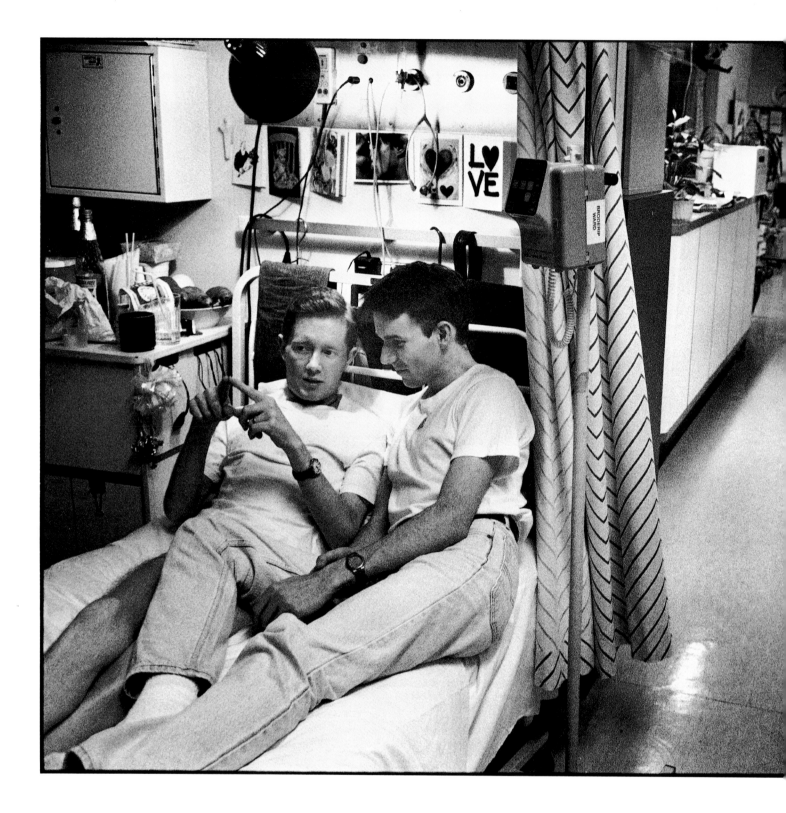

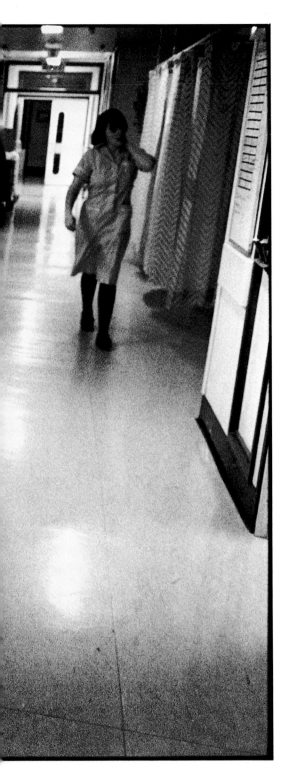

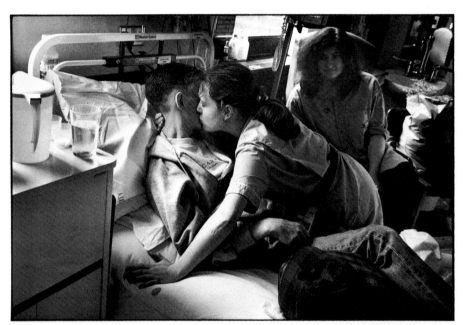

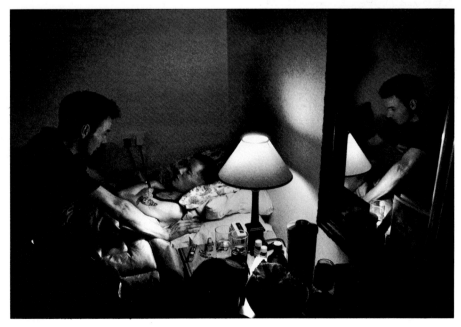

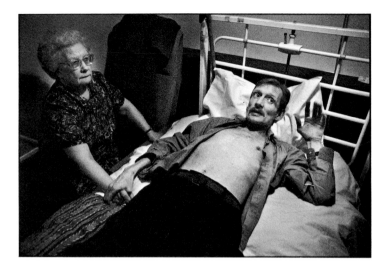

Ian

With a Portacath implanted in his chest, Ian learns to puncture his skin to inject medication through the implant direct to a main vein. Watched by his mother, he practises the difficult and painful procedure, and at the end of the week becomes independent enough to return home.

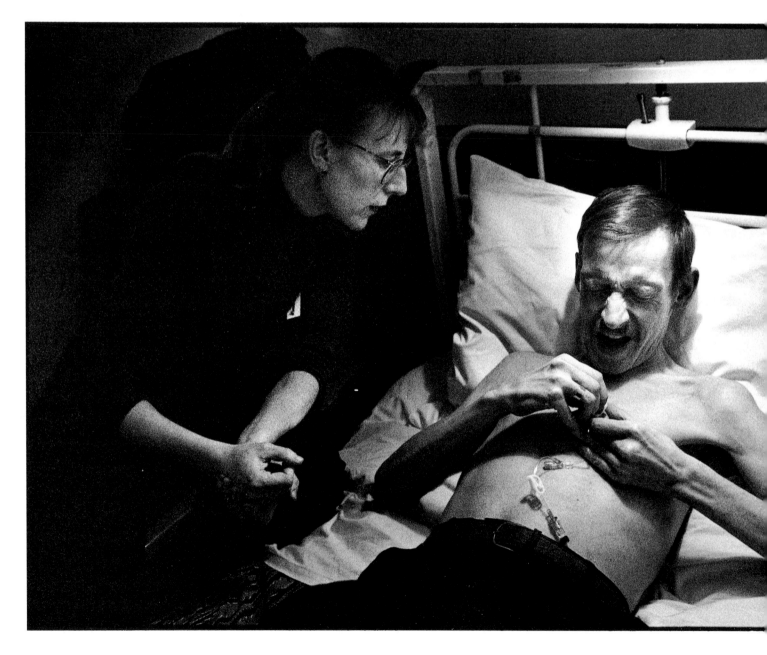

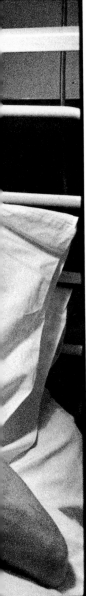
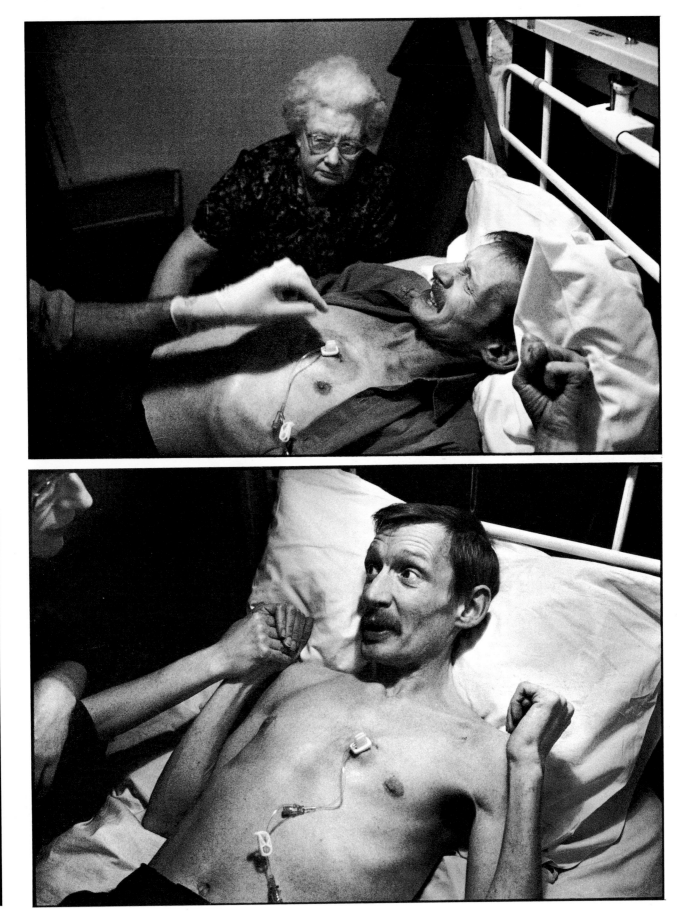

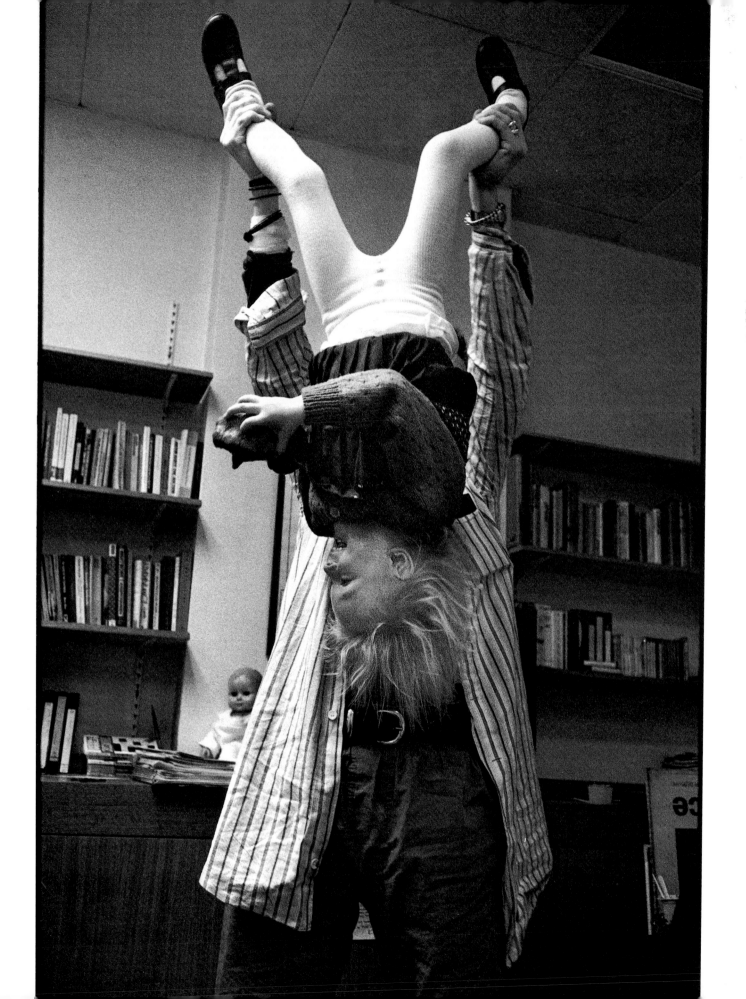

Steven

The ward held no fears for Steven, who described it to his frequent visitors as his 'West End Hotel.' Steven tried to maintain control over his treatment and often challenged the medical team at the hospital about his prescriptions and blood transfusions.

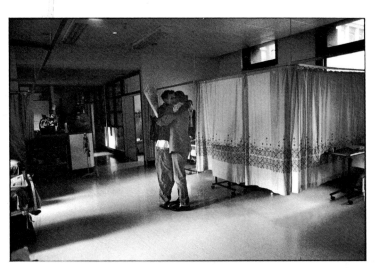

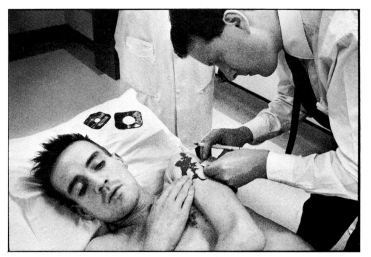

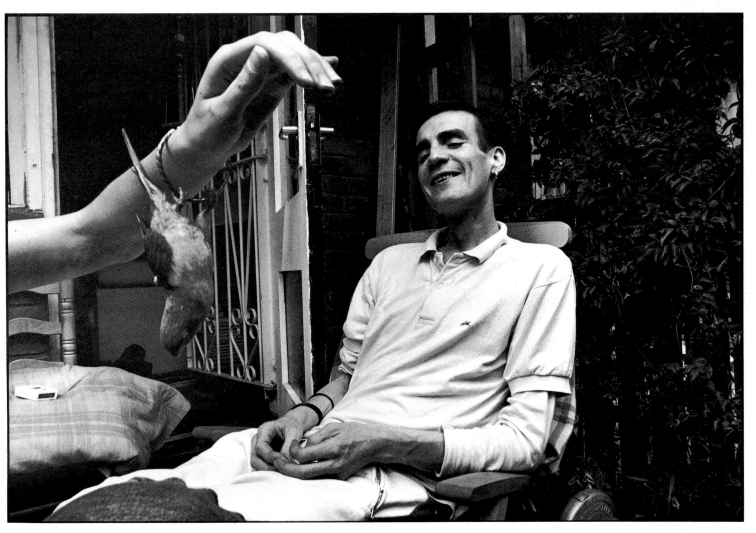

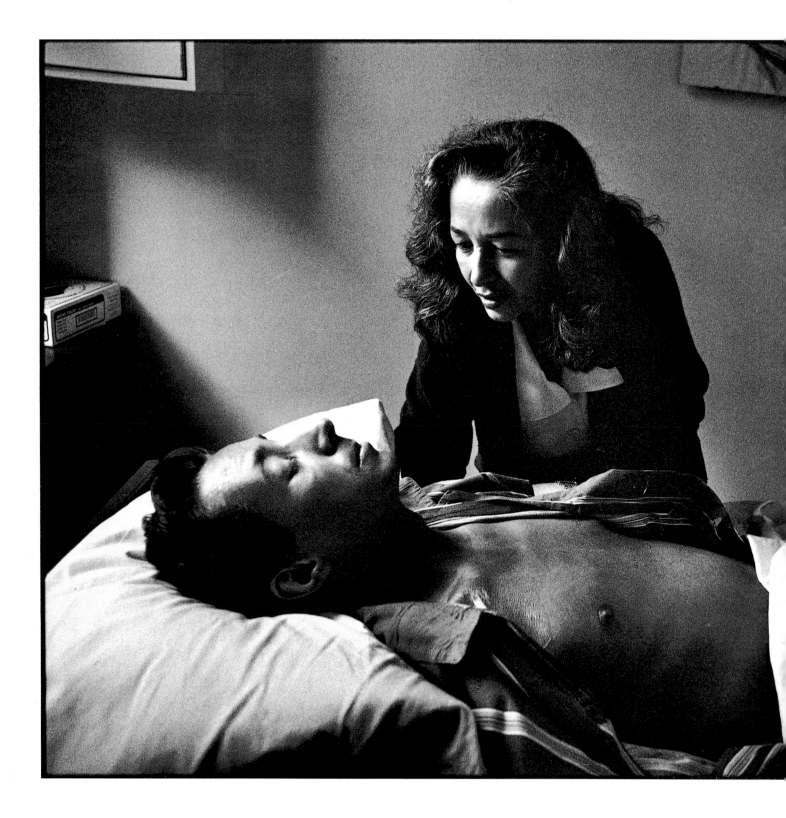

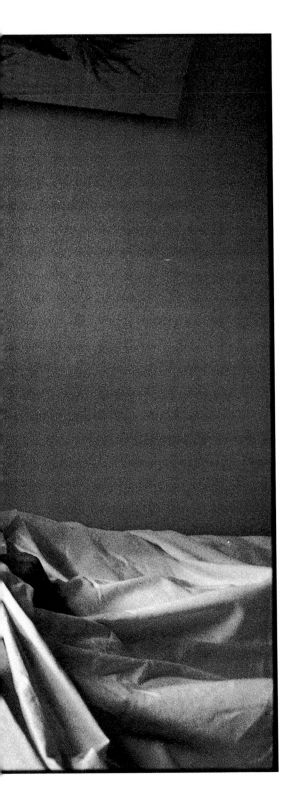

André

André was in for routine treatment when he suddenly became critically ill. With his mother and his partner at his side he seemed about to die when, just as suddenly, he revived, and recuperated with astonishing speed.

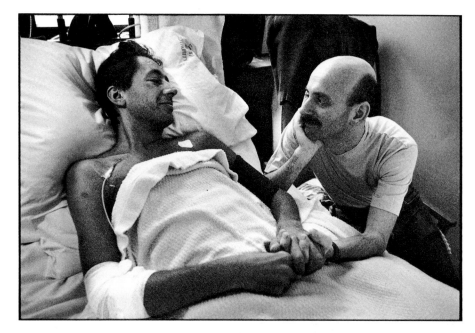

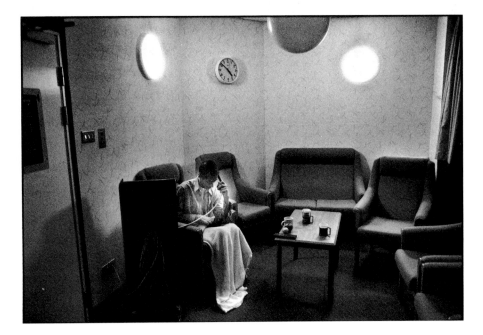

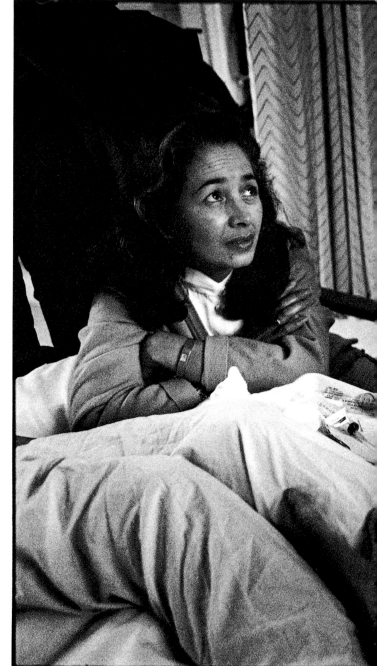

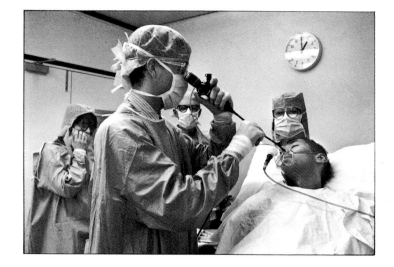

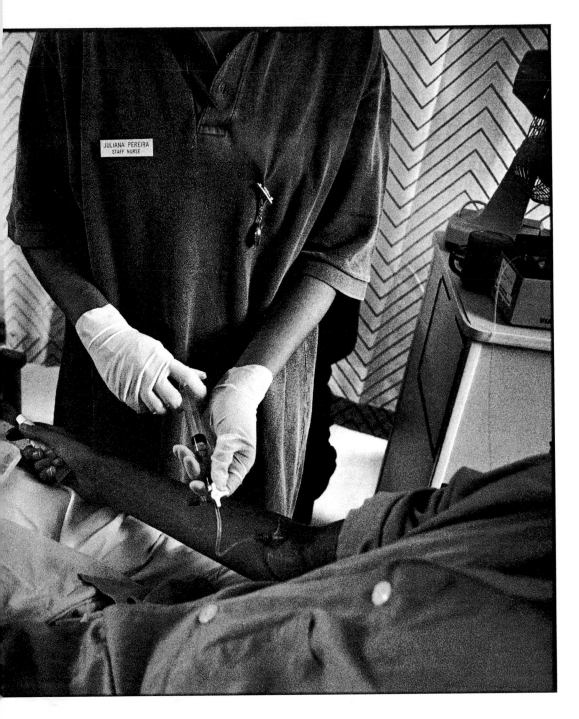

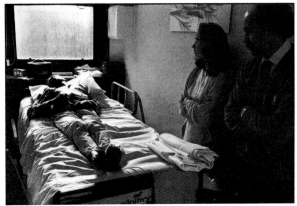

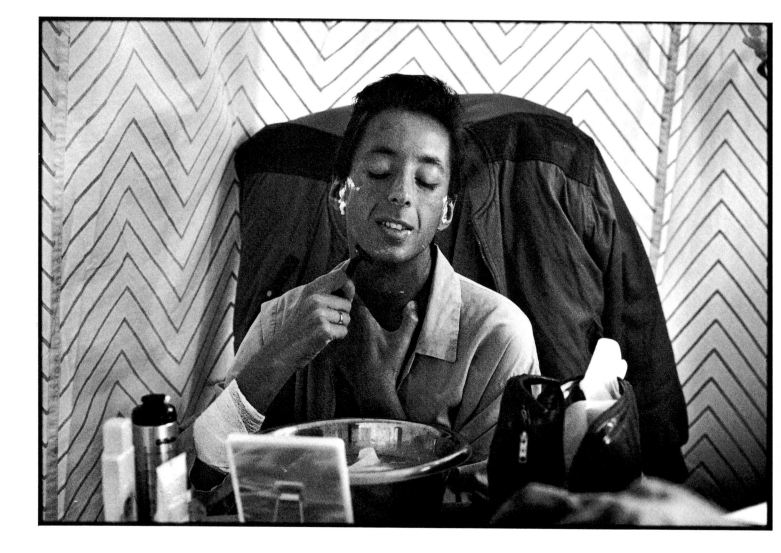

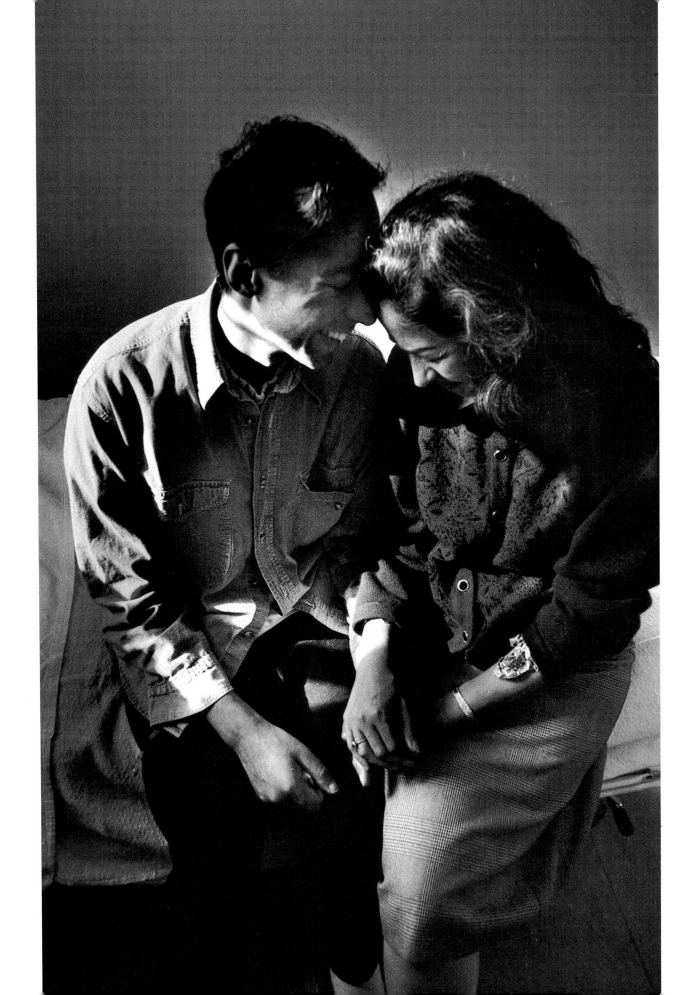

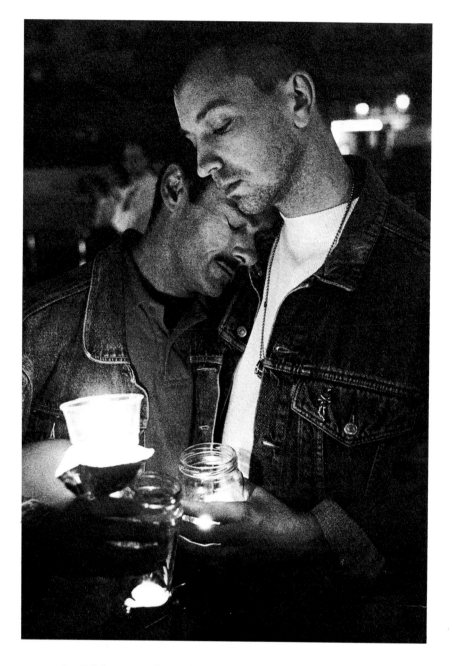

Candlelight Memorial at Trafalgar Square, London, May 1993. In memory of those who have died with AIDS. *Photograph by Mark Power.*